BASIC HEALTH
PUBLICATIONS
USER'S GUIDE

TO PYCNOGENOL®, NATURE'S MOST VERSATILE SUPPLEMENT

Learn How to Use This Remarkable
Supplement to Fight
Inflammation and Reinvigorate
Your Total Health.

RICHARD A. PASSWATER, PH.D.
JACK CHALLEM Series Editor

The information contained in this book is based upon the research and personal and professional experiences of the author. It is not intended as a substitute for consulting with your physician or other healthcare provider. Any attempt to diagnose and treat an illness should be done under the direction of a healthcare professional.

The publisher does not advocate the use of any particular healthcare protocol but believes the information in this book should be available to the public. The publisher and author are not responsible for any adverse effects or consequences resulting from the use of the suggestions, preparations, or procedures discussed in this book. Should the reader have any questions concerning the appropriateness of any procedures or preparations mentioned, the author and the publisher strongly suggest consulting a professional healthcare advisor.

Series Editor: Jack Challem
Editor: Tara Durkin
Typesetter: Gary A. Rosenberg
Series Cover Designer: Mike Stromberg

Basic Health Publications User's Guides are published by Basic Health Publications, Inc.
28812 Top of the World Drive
Laguna Beach, CA 92651
949-715-7327

Printed in the United States of America

10   9   8   7   6   5   4   3   2

Contents

INTRODUCTION

If you could take a single natural product that would not only reduce your risk of heart disease and protect and improve your cardiovascular and circulation systems, but would also reduce inflammation, protect your skin against wrinkling, and reduce your risk of more than sixty diseases, would you take it? Of course you would. Any reasonable person would, provided he or she is aware of the product's strong scientific background.

The one natural product that offers all of these benefits, and more, is a natural extract from the bark of French maritime pine trees. It's called Pycnogenol (pronounced pick-nah-jeh-nol), and a growing body of scientific research and physicians' experiences proves that it can have a profoundly important effect on your health. Clinical studies involving more than 3,000 people have confirmed what many people have known for some time: Pycnogenol works.

In this book, I will introduce you to the health benefits of Pycnogenol. I first learned about Pycnogenol in the late 1980s at a nutrition conference. Charles Haimoff, a German chemist who was the chief executive of Horphag Research Ltd., showed me the research his company had conducted up to that time and introduced me to several European professors at their University laboratories so that they might share their research with me. I became very interested and soon began my own research and writing about Pycnogenol. My first article appeared in 1991. I find that the body of science involving Pycnogenol grows so rapidly that I feel compelled to bring new information to the public on a regular basis so that they might benefit from the ongoing research.

CHAPTER 1

HOW PYCNOGENOL WORKS TO OPTIMIZE YOUR HEALTH

The story of Pycnogenol goes back hundreds of years. Pycnogenol evolved from the pine bark and pine needle potion of Native North American medicine men. It was used to treat conditions now recognized as scurvy due to vitamin C deficiency, yet it is not a rich source of vitamin C itself. It is, however, a source of other nutrients, several of which recycle antioxidant nutrients such as vitamin C.

Antioxidants
Antioxidants protect against the unwanted, disease-causing reactions of oxygen.

Scientific interest in this pine bark and pine needle tonic was stimulated by reports from Jacques Cartier's French expedition to Canada in 1535 to find a northwest passage to China. During the winter, the frozen Hudson Bay caused the expedition to stop at the Native American villages of Stadacona and Hochelaga. Because the explorers had to spend the entire winter there, they exhausted their supply of fresh foods. They soon developed scurvy.

Scurvy had already killed twenty-five members of the expedition, and fifty more were seriously ill, by the time Cartier befriended a local Native American, Chief Domagaia. The chief prepared a decoction from what was described as a conifer believed to have been pine. The bark and needles were boiled to make a tea that was drunk several times a day. The men recovered within a week or two after beginning the treatment. They didn't understand how the decoction worked at the time, but it was due to the fact that the pine needles supplied a small amount of vitamin C and the pine bark supplied vitamin C–enhancing bioflavonoids.

Scientists aware of the historical accounts of Cartier's expedition became intrigued. They wanted to find out why a tree bark extract cured the explorers of scurvy.

Fruit acids
Small organic acids found in foods, including various fruits, vegetables, nuts, seeds, and beans.

In 1970, with the advent of better analytical instruments and funding from Horphag Research Ltd., it was determined that pine bark extract was a defined mixture of fruit acids and procyanidins. In 1984, G. Pirasteh, Ph.D., and Peter Rohdewald, Ph.D., identified and quantified most of the ingredients.

Not only does Pycnogenol have a long and colorful history, it has proven its value over decades

**Procyanidins
(proanthocyanidins)**
A class of bioflavonoids. About 250 have been identified in nature. They are named after the blue hue they give to plants ("cyano" means dark blue).

of commercial use with millions of consumers around the world. It has made a significant difference in the health of these people. Through the years, the commercial extraction process used to produce Pycnogenol has been patented, as have uses of Pycnogenol for several health conditions. These include the use

of this unique extract as an antioxidant (U.S. Patent No. 4,698,360, granted on October 6, 1987), for improving blood circulation and reducing the risk of heart attacks by improving the condition of blood platelets (U.S. Patent No. 5,720,956, granted on February 24, 1998), for treating dysmenorrhea and endometriosis (U.S. Patent No. 6,372,266, granted on April 16, 2002), and for treating erectile dysfunction (impotence) (U.S. Patent No. 6,565,851, granted on May 20, 2003). There have been 140 articles about Pycnogenol published in the scientific and medical journals and more than 3,000 people have been the subjects of clinical studies.

Nutrient or Herb, or Both?

Some may consider Pycnogenol an herb and others may consider it a nutrient complex. Both are correct, but my more-than-fifteen-years experience with Pycnogenol research leads me to consider Pycnogenol primarily as a nutrient complex.

Before it was recognized that many of Pycnogenol's health benefits were due to its unique complex of nutrient bioflavonoids, it was used more or less as an herbal remedy or over-the-counter treatment for hay fever and swelling of the ankles and legs. As more and more people used Pycnogenol for a single ailment, they soon recognized that it was also good for other purposes. It was later found to be a superantioxidant and nutrient.

Scientists and physicians continually learn of additional health benefits as more and more people use Pycnogenol. After the nutrient was introduced in Europe as a product to help nourish capillaries (small blood vessels) and skin— as suggested by the research on bioflavonoids by Nobel Laureate Dr. Albert Szent-Györgyi—European physicians discovered that Pycnogenol did much more. With use, it was discovered that Pycnogenol was also a natural cure for hay fever.

Bioflavonoids
A class of thousands of beneficial compounds found in plants. They have a host of beneficial effects including being antioxidants.

Through the years, research has shown that Pycnogenol increases capillary resistance by protecting the major skin protein collagen and the ground substance between the cells. This was part of the explanation as to why a pine bark decoction used by Native North Americans cured scurvy. In scurvy, blood leaks out of the capillaries to virtually drown the victims in their own blood. Further research with Pycnogenol and capillaries confirmed that it improves microcirculation by both improving capillary strength and improving blood cell flexibility. Soon it was also learned that Pycnogenol improves skin by reducing the degradation of the skin proteins collagen and elastin.

It was not until 1987 that a patent was issued for Pycnogenol's strong antioxidant effect that protects so well against harmful free radicals. Although Pycnogenol was available in Europe for many years, it was not introduced as a dietary supplement in the United States until 1987. At the beginning of the 1990s, the general population was beginning to learn of the health benefits of antioxidants. As more people learned of the antioxidant power of Pycnogenol, they also learned of its other health benefits. Slowly but surely, Pycnogenol's benefits became known as one helped person told another, and today it is one of the most popular dietary supplements.

Researchers in the United States have become very interested in Pycnogenol. Beginning in 1995, U.S. scientists started publishing research reports showing that Pycnogenol regenerates vitamin C, protects against stress and smoking risk factors involved in heart disease and stroke, reduces stress-induced increases in blood pressure, protects against Syndrome X and type 2 diabetes, improves the immune system, and much more.

Why the Strange Name?

The Native North Americans did not call this pine bark extract "Pycnogenol." This was a name coined later after many years of scientific study and standardization of the extraction process, and the determination of one species of pine tree as the best source. This species is the maritime pine from Landes de Gascogne, commonly called the French maritime pine tree. Its formal scientific name is the *Pinus pinaster*, subspecies *atlantica*. However, it is also referred to in the scientific literature as Atlantic pine, *Pinus maritima,* Pin des Landes, *Pinus pinaster* Sol., and *Pinus pinaster* Aiton. Regardless of the different names, it is the only species that grows in the 4,000 square miles of forest along the Bay of Biscay (Atlantic Ocean), situated between the vineyards of Bordeaux to the north and the Pyrenees mountains to the south.

The name "Pycnogenol" was selected because it reflects the fact that many of the nutrient bioflavonoids in the extract are made by joining together smaller bioflavonoids. The larger bioflavonoid molecules, which chemists call oligomeric procyanidins, are formed when nature joins together two or more of the smaller bioflavonoid molecules, catechin and/or epicatechin. The word "pycnogenol" was taken from the Greek root word "pycno," meaning to condense or thicken. (Chemists refer to the process of joining smaller molecules into large one "condensation reactions" or "polymerization.") The "gen" portion of the word is from "generate," and "ol" represents the chemical class (family). This suggests that this blend of bioflavonoids contains large molecules that have been joined together from small molecules.

Now the name is trademarked. The U.S. Patent and Trademark Office issued a trademark to Horphag Research Ltd. for the name "Pycnogenol" for dietary and nutritional supplements on May 11, 1993 (Reg. No. 1,769,633). An official logo depicting a pine tree encircled with the words "Pycnogenol French Maritime Pine Bark Extract" is often used on products and advertisements.

Pycnogenol is also a registered trade name in more than ninety other countries, including Australia, Brazil, India, Italy, Singapore, Spain, and the United Kingdom.

How Pycnogenol Works

This section offers an overview of how Pycnogenol

works—more detailed explanations follow in later chapters. Pycnogenol works for a number of reasons. First, it's a natural complex of several powerful antioxidants—that is, substances that protect your body from free radicals and the ravages of the aging process. Antioxidants and free radicals are explained in Chapter 2.

Second, it contains unique compounds that have specific interactions with several body systems, especially in optimizing nitric oxide balance. Nitric oxide is covered in Chapter 4.

Third, it contains many of the beneficial compounds found in fruits and vegetables, but it concentrates them so you benefit from higher potencies. Pycnogenol is somewhat like a natural herbal remedy, but it has a long track record of exceptional safety.

A brief summary of Pycnogenol's biochemical actions follows:

1. It terminates free radicals, thus protecting cells.

2. It enhances immune function.

3. It binds to the skin proteins collagen and elastin to protect tissue and to seal leaky capillaries.

4. It improves the functioning of blood vessels, large and small, from arteries to the microcirculation of capillaries.

5. It inhibits tiny blood cells from sticking together to cause circulation problems such as heart attack, stroke, and deep vein thrombosis.

These five biochemical actions produce dozens of health benefits including:

- Protection against dangerous molecules known as free radicals, which speed up the aging process and set the stage for heart disease, cancer, and more than sixty other diseases.

- Stronger blood vessel walls, which protects the

linings of blood vessels and reduces edema.

- Improved circulation and maintained slipperiness of blood cells, which helps prevent heart attack–causing blood clots from forming.

- Protection against stress.

- A strengthened immune system.

- Relaxing of blood vessels, which improves blood circulation and helps to normalize blood pressure.

- Reduced inflammation, which improves joint flexibility.

- Relief from hay fever and allergies.

- Reduction of menstrual disorders.

- Smooth and youthfully flexible skin.

- Abnormal pigmentation of the skin is counteracted.

- Protection against the complications of diabetes such as retinopathy.

- Improved learning ability and memory retention.

- Reduced risk of cataracts.

- Improved healing.

- The biochemical actions of Pycnogenol can help to overcome attention deficit hyperactive disorder (ADHD, or hyperactivity).

After seeing the long list of health benefits, you might wonder how could one supplement possibly do so much? To some, it might sound like a "cure all" or "snake oil," unless they understand that the many health benefits are achieved through a few basic actions. Some of the nutrients, such as the antioxidants, affect many body systems and thus are factors in preventing many diseases.

Antioxidants are involved in reducing the risk of

more than sixty diseases. The action of Pycnogenol in boosting the immune system explains how it increases protection against many infections.

Another part of the answer is that Pycnogenol is not just one nutrient. Since it contains so many nutrients, it has several different actions. Most of the compounds act chiefly as antioxidants, while others block the actions of undesirable compounds in the body.

In later chapters of this book, we will examine the research that shows that Pycnogenol is a powerful and effective antioxidant and anti-inflammatory nutrient, that it improves blood circulation and makes skin healthier and younger looking. For now, here is a brief overview of the research on this important dietary supplement.

Research has been carried out on Pycnogenol since 1965. However, these data have been retained as unpublished internal research reports of Horphag Research Ltd., the company that developed Pycnogenol. Extensive safety studies have been carried out under the direction of Dr. Peter Rohdewald of the University of Munster in Germany. Research on capillary health has been conducted by Dr. Miklos Gabor of the Szent-Györgyi Medical University in Hungary. Studies on Pycnogenol protection of skin have been carried out by Dr. Antti Arstila of the University of Jyvaeskylae in Finland.

More recent research has centered on Pycnogenol's effects on heart disease, the immune system, attention deficit disorder, and Alzheimer's disease. Ronald Watson, Ph.D., of the University of Arizona, Tucson, has been researching Pycnogenol's action in boosting the immune system, protecting against sunburn, improving hypertension, and protecting against heart disease. Dr. Lester Packer of the University of California, Berkeley, studied how Pycnogenol functions as an antioxidant, how it protects nerve cells, and how it acts as an anti-inflammatory agent (see review by Packer et al., 1999, listed in Selected References).

Dr. Schubert of the Salk Institute has studied how Pycnogenol helps protect against Alzheimer's disease. Dr. Benjamin Lau of Loma Linda University has discovered that Pycnogenol enhances antioxidant defenses of body cells and improves learning ability and memory retention.

Dr. Lau and his colleagues have also found that Pycnogenol compensates for the age-related decline of the immune system. They have further shown that Pycnogenol inhibits generation of inflammatory mediators in the inflammatory cells.

Dr. T. Kohama, a Japanese gynecologist, showed Pycnogenol's benefits for menstrual disorders. Dr I. (Ken) Jialal and his colleagues at the University of Texas at Dallas demonstrated that the blood of volunteers who took Pycnogenol had a significantly increased antioxidant capacity.

Professors Arcangeli and Spartera of the University of Aquila, Italy, in independent clinical studies have shown beneficial effects of Pycnogenol in chronic venous insufficiency. Professor Balestrazzi from the same university showed Pycnogenol's benefits in diabetic retinopathy.

As the number of scientific publications increase, there will be additional scientists eager to research the health benefits of Pycnogenol.

Why Pycnogenol Is Unique

Pycnogenol is a unique supplement. Although many different companies sell Pycnogenol, it comes from only one source. The makers of some other products may claim benefits similar to those of Pycnogenol, but there is only one product—patent protected—that is extracted from French maritime pine trees and provides this unique complex of nutrients.

Many of the procyanidin bioflavonoids of Pycnogenol are specific to it because they come from a unique plant. However, Pycnogenol contains other procyanidins and organic acids that are also found in a broad range of fruits and vegetables, as well as some herbs. For example, sorghum, avocado, strawberries, bananas, and grapes contain various procyanidins. Caffeic acid and ferulic acid are found in parsley and spinach. Onions contain caffeic acid, and rhubarb and grapes contain ferulic acid. Gallic acid is found in eggplant and radish. However, nowhere else in nature are Pycnogenol's specific procyanidins and unique blend of bioflavonoid nutrients found.

The importance of Pycnogenol's distinctive combination of procyanidins and organic acids has been demonstrated by studies in which Pycnogenol was chemically and physically divided into smaller fractions according to their molecular sizes. One fraction contained a range of compounds having the smallest molecular sizes. Another fraction contained various compounds with the largest molecular sizes, and the third fraction contained a range of the intermediate-sized molecules. While one fraction showed superiority in one action or another, the benefits of the individual fractions never equaled the benefits of the complete blend.

The many diverse nutrients in Pycnogenol result in synergy unmatched by any other known blend of nutrients. The smaller molecules provide antioxidant activity more quickly and can penetrate smaller cellular compartments, the larger molecules provide longer-lasting as well as more diverse actions. Together, this combination provides effects not demonstrated by any other dietary supplement.

One of the advantages of the precise extraction method used to make Pycnogenol is that it produces a consistent nutrient makeup, which is necessary for clinical studies and clinical use. Scientists stress that it is important for products used clinically to be consistent from batch to batch and year to year. Just think of the medical chaos that would ensue if one batch of penicillin tablets contained twice the amount of penicillin of the next batch. Or if the potency of aspirin varied from batch to batch.

It is difficult to find natural products that are consistent from crop to crop. The nutrient content of wheat and corn vary according to the season and the soil. Herbs also vary depending on the source. Pycnogenol is a natural product that comes from a single species. The bark of the maritime pine grows over the twenty-five-year-plus lifetime of the tree and varies little in bioflavonoid content. In contrast to this, other natural products such as grapes vary from region to region and crop to crop, as do the wines produced from them. Doctors can't conduct meaningful studies with medicines or nutrients that may have been from a "vintage year."

Besides being from a single species that grows over decades in the same region, Pycnogenol is extracted by a very controlled process and standardized when dried to a powder to produce a product that is always consistent.

CHAPTER 2

UNDERSTANDING THE ANTIOXIDANT POWER OF PYCNOGENOL

In Chapter 1, I mentioned how difficult it is for people to accept the fact that Pycnogenol can do so much, unless they understand why and how it works. I explained that the many health benefits of Pycnogenol are achieved through a few basic actions. Now is a good time to look at one of these mechanisms in more detail to better understand how Pycnogenol can prevent and/or alleviate so many diseases and disorders.

The strong antioxidant capability of Pycnogenol alone offers protection against more than sixty diseases that involve free radicals. Free radicals are harmful molecules that damage the body. You can think of free radicals as biological terrorists. Quite simply, they can be bad for your health.

In chemistry, atoms that are found grouped together can be called a "radical." This group or radical generally stays together during a chemical reaction and can be transferred from molecule to molecule.

> **Free radicals**
> *Unstable, high-energy molecules that damage the body. Free-radical damage disrupts normal biochemistry and leads to many diseases.*

Sometimes during very high energy chemical reactions, radicals can have an electron pulled away, causing the group to temporarily break free from the molecule. When this happens, it is called a "free radical." While this unstable, high-energy fragment is free, its energy forces attract an electron from another molecule. A free radical can pull an electron from most biological compounds, thus restoring its original electron content, but causing the other compound that has lost an electron to itself become a free radical.

This free-radical reaction can perpetuate until a key biological molecule becomes permanently damaged. Scientists have estimated that each cell in your body (and you have billions of cells) suffers 10,000 free-radical "hits" each day. The amount of damage depends on how well the cell is protected by antioxidants. The higher your levels of antioxidants, the greater the amount of protection.

Free radicals damage cell membranes, cellular proteins, DNA, RNA, and other essential body components, disrupting normal biochemistry and leading to many diseases. Free radicals can be the sole cause of a few diseases but more often are involved in the disease process by predisposing the human body to diseases directly caused by other factors. Free radicals also may worsen existing conditions and antagonize the healing process.

First, let's look at the free-radical-related health conditions or diseases that involve more than one organ. These are aging, including disorders of "premature aging" and immune deficiency of aging; cancer; inflammatory immune injury, including nutritional deficiencies, alcohol damage, and radiation injury, reproductive disorders, and abnormal sperm morphology.

Then there are the free-radical-related diseases that involve a primary single organ. These are blood cell disorders, including systemic lupus erythematosus and sickle-cell anemia; lung disorders, including asthma, cigarette smoke–induced effects, emphysema, hyperoxia, bronchopulmonary dysphasia, cystic fibrosis, disorders caused by oxidant pollutants, acute respiratory distress syndrome (ARDS); heart and cardiovascular system disorders, including atherosclerosis (via oxidation of LDL), heart attack (acute myocardial infarction via coronary thrombosis via platelet aggregation), endothelial injury, vasospasms, and kidney disorders; gastrointestinal tract and liver disorders, including hepatitis, endotoxin liver injury, joint abnormalities, and rheumatoid arthritis; brain disorders, including those caused by neurotoxins, senile dementia, Parkinson's disease, Alzheimer's disease, stroke (thrombosis in cerebral vessels), cerebral trauma from stroke (hypertensive cerebrovascular injury); eye disorders, including cataracts, macular degeneration, ocular hemorrhage, degenerative retinal damage, diabetic retinopathy, and photic retinopathy; skin disorders, including melasma (chloasma), sunburn (solar radiation), burn (thermal injury), psoriasis, and dental diseases such as periodontitis. There are more free-radical-related diseases, but I think you get the idea.

As will be explained in later chapters, free radicals are involved in cardiovascular diseases and other chronic degenerate diseases. Free radicals also accelerate the aging process, and as a result are involved in decreasing our defenses against germs. Arthritis, Alzheimer's disease, and Parkinson's disease are also linked to free radicals, and studies indicate that antioxidants likely reduce the risk of these diseases.

Antioxidants

Antioxidants protect against free radicals and the unwanted reactions of oxygen. Oxygen is a very reactive element, which is why it rusts iron, promotes combustion, and supports the life process. Iron and iron-containing objects that are left out in air (which contains oxygen) rust, or as chemists say, "oxidize." The process by which things react with oxygen is called oxidation. A substance that prevents or slows the oxidation process is called an antioxidant. Antioxidants also protect other substances, such as living tissue, against damage caused by oxygen.

In the body, it's important for oxygen to be

channeled into the right places and kept away from other places. We don't want oxygen to react with vital cell components. This would damage them much like rust damages iron. In the body, unwanted oxidation of cell components can set the stage for aging, heart disease, cancer, and many other chronic degenerative diseases. Antioxidants sacrifice themselves to protect vital components. As a powerful antioxidant that also helps recharge other antioxidants, Pycnogenol helps protect us against the damage of free radicals very effectively and thus helps protect us from the more than sixty diseases associated with free radicals.

To qualify as an antioxidant, a few good molecules must protect many, many other molecules by neutralizing bad molecules or fragments of molecules. Our bodies make some antioxidants. However, we are dependent on the diet to supply many antioxidants. Important antioxidant nutrients include vitamins, minerals, amino acids, and coenzymes.

Minerals are not direct antioxidants, but several minerals can become vital components of antioxidant enzymes made by the body. Such minerals include selenium, which is needed to make the antioxidant enzyme glutathione peroxidase; iron, which is needed for catalase; and manganese, copper, and zinc, which are needed to make superoxide dismutase. (Incidentally, Pycnogenol contains small amounts of all these minerals.)

Sulfur compounds, such as the sulfur-containing amino acids cysteine and methionine, help the body produce the most common antioxidant within cells, glutathione.

Antioxidant coenzymes, such as nicotinamide adenine dinucleotide (NADH), coenzyme Q_{10}, and alpha-lipoic acid, can be made in the body as well as obtained in the diet.

Bioflavonoids

Bioflavonoids are antioxidant compounds that can

partially replace the need for vitamin C in specific biochemical reactions and, thus, save some vitamin C. Early research by Nobel Laureate Dr. Albert Szent-Györgyi suggested that bioflavonoids had additional properties that justified their classification as vitamins. American scientists have rejected this view, but many European scientists believe that bioflavonoids are at least semi-essential and that the vitamin hypothesis merits further study.

Bioflavonoids, often called flavonoids, are a class of thousands of beneficial compounds found in plants. The structures of these antioxidant compounds enables them to easily donate electrons to other molecules. This ability to donate electrons, a type of subatomic particle, is a characteristic of all antioxidants. There are thousands of bioflavonoids existing in nature. Scientists have identified over 4,000 of them, but they are sure that there are several thousand more yet to be discovered.

Flavonoids are found in fruits, vegetables, nuts, seeds, grains, cacao, and in beverages such as tea and wine. Many flavonoids are pigments that provide several fruits with their blue and purple colors as well as some of the reds and emerald green.

In addition to their antioxidant properties, bioflavonoids have a host of other beneficial effects in the body. Studies have shown that bioflavonoids possess antiviral, anti-inflammatory, antihistamine, and even anticarcinogenic properties.

The Antioxidant Power of Pycnogenol

Pycnogenol contains very powerful organic antioxidants such as the relatively large molecules of the procyanidins (bioflavonoids) and the relatively small molecules of catechin, epicatechin, and organic acids. The large array of molecular size in the numerous antioxidants allow antioxidants to reach cell interiors as well as circulate in the bloodstream to protect cell exteriors, destroying free radicals before they can do damage to body components.

Not only does Pycnogenol contain potent organic antioxidants and measurable levels of the inorganic minerals the body needs to build antioxidant enzymes, it also increases the levels of these antioxidant enzymes and related antioxidants within the cells. Dr. Z. H. Wei and his colleagues from Loma Linda University in California have shown that Pycnogenol can double the concentration of superoxide dismutase, catalase, and glutathione.

An important reason why Pycnogenol is such a potent antioxidant is that it is a natural mixture of several types of antioxidants, so it distributes antioxidant nutrients widely throughout the body. The Pycnogenol complex of antioxidants provides compounds of varying sizes that can function effectively in different regions of the body over varying periods of time.

The larger procyanidins are very effective in the bloodstream, whereas the smaller flavonoid molecules and organic acids can readily enter cell interiors. The large oligomeric procyanidins have several points in their molecules that can annihilate free radicals. Vitamin E, in contrast, has only one such point. The free-radical annihilating points are called phenolic groups, and vitamin E is a monophenol, whereas Pycnogenol is a polyphenol.

The various nutrients in Pycnogenol have chemical structures that protect against different types of free radicals. Whereas a single antioxidant compound, such as vitamin E or vitamin C, is protective against several specific kinds of free radicals, a mixture of many different types of antioxidants protects against a greater range of free radicals. Its unique position is caused by its ability to double the content of antioxidative enzymes inside the cell, in addition to directly neutralizing free radicals.

Pycnogenol Regenerates Other Antioxidants

One of the reasons that antioxidants work together

synergistically is that some antioxidants can regenerate other antioxidants. For example, Pycnogenol can regenerate "used" or "spent" vitamin C, which in turn, can regenerate used vitamin E. This means that Pycnogenol enables the sparse amounts of vitamin C and vitamin E found in most diets to function as if there were higher levels in the diet. This is a result of recharging the spent vitamins to work again instead of being removed from the body.

When vitamin E or vitamin C molecules come into contact with free radicals, they donate an electron to the free radical, making it a normal nonreactive molecule. This causes the vitamin E or vitamin C molecule to become a weak free radical. This weak free radical does no harm to the body, but since it has given up an electron itself, it can no longer stop free-radical reactions. Thus, the vitamin E radicals or vitamin C radicals are useless; the body usually destroys them by breaking them apart into smaller compounds to permit their removal from the body via the kidneys.

On the other hand, if the inactive vitamin C radical comes into contact with one of the bioflavonoids in Pycnogenol, it can be regenerated back into active vitamin C. Active vitamin C can also regenerate an inactive vitamin E radical. This effect of Pycnogenol is possible because the larger procyanidin molecules in Pycnogenol stabilize the lifetime of the inactive vitamin C radical so that it doesn't decompose and leave the body; instead, it can last long enough to capture its missing electron from one of the many molecules of the procyanidins.

Pycnogenol May Be the Most Powerful Antioxidant Nutrient

Pycnogenol is the best of the many antioxidants that Dr. Lester Packer and his colleagues at the University of California, Berkeley, studied for their effectiveness against free radicals in 1997.

According to the studies by Dr. Packer's group,

Pycnogenol is the most powerful antioxidant complex that has been widely studied under identical laboratory conditions and reported in the scientific literature. This includes even the more widely known antioxidant nutrients, vitamins C and E. Furthermore, as just discussed, Pycnogenol recycles these vitamins back into their protective antioxidant forms.

Dr. M. Chida and his colleagues at the University of Tokyo carried out a study to compare the ability of different antioxidants to protect retinal lipids (fats in the eye retina) from damage by free radicals. They found that Pycnogenol was far more potent than vitamins C and E, lipoic acid, coenzyme Q_{10}, and grape seed extract. Pycnogenol was six times better than grape seed extract, nine times better than vitamin E, and many orders of magnitude better than coenzyme Q_{10}, vitamin C, and lipoic acid.

In addition, Dr. Benjamin Lau of Loma Linda University has found that Pycnogenol stimulates production of endogenous antioxidants within cells.

When the several studies of Pycnogenol's antioxidant capabilities are considered together, they indicate that Pycnogenol may be the most powerful scavenger of oxygen and nitrogen free radicals, as well as other reactive oxygen species (ROS) and reactive nitrogen species (RNS). Pycnogenol has been shown to be the strongest scavenger of hydroxyl free radicals and superoxide anion radicals among compounds and extracts tested.

When comparing antioxidants, several factors must be looked at. One antioxidant may be better retained in one body organ or system than in another. Or an antioxidant may be more efficient against one type of free radical than it is against another. The only fair way to compare antioxidants is to compare their profiles of actions against various free radicals.

An important factor is how well the various

antioxidant nutrients are absorbed. Dr. Kenny Jialal of the University of Texas has measured the antioxidant capacity of Pycnogenol in volunteers and has found that the total protective effect (measured as ORAC) of Pycnogenol in the blood increases dramatically soon after taking the supplement. This shows that Pycnogenol is highly bioavailable and provides considerable antioxidant protection.

There may not be just one antioxidant nutrient that is the best in all possible systems—but Pycnogenol appears to be the most powerful in the most systems, especially of the systems of major importance.

The Antioxidant Team

The fact that Pycnogenol is a powerful and versatile antioxidant does not mean that it is the only antioxidant that you should take as a supplement. Many antioxidant nutrients work together as a team. Some simple antioxidants, such as vitamin C and vitamin E, are essential to life and must be part of the diet to maintain life.

Others, such as coenzyme Q_{10}, alpha-lipoic acid, and NADH, can be made in the body and are not dietary essential even though they are also involved in metabolism. These antioxidant nutrients have specific roles that are not replaced by other antioxidants. However, they can be readily consumed by free-radical reactions, and they are not abundant in the diet.

Pycnogenol has sparing action on vitamin C and can regenerate used vitamin C. Vitamin C can, in turn, recycle used vitamin E. Vitamin E is fat-soluble and dwells in the body in fat-friendly areas, such as cell membranes and lipoproteins. Vitamin C and the bioflavonoids of Pycnogenol are water soluble and dwell in water-compatible areas such as the bloodstream and cell interiors.

Although Pycnogenol is not considered to be a dietary essential nutrient, it should be included in the daily diet because it is a powerful antioxidant that has many additional health benefits.

Pycnogenol: More Than an Antioxidant

Pycnogenol is much more than a powerful, multi-purpose antioxidant. It also has strong anti-inflammatory, immune boosting, spasmolytic (antispasmodic), and anticoagulant (anti–blood clotting) actions.

In addition, Pycnogenol helps balance and control the production of nitric oxide, which is a good compound in the artery linings and certain other areas but can be a very harmful compound otherwise. We will discuss nitric oxide later in Chapter 4.

Pycnogenol also stimulates production of skin protein and binds to skin proteins to protect them against harmful enzymes. We will look into this further in Chapter 5.

All of these actions combine to make Pycnogenol unique in its ability to give significant health benefits not known to be produced by any other antioxidant nutrient.

CHAPTER 3

HEALTHY AGING

There is no physical or mental condition directly attributed to the passage of time. It is not the passage of time that ages us, it is the accumulation of deleterious chemical events that deteriorates our bodies into the condition we call aged. Some of the diseases or disorders associated with aging can also occur in the young. Children can have cancer, high blood pressure, arthritis, and the like, so it is not simply the number of years that ages us. What, then, is aging?

Aging is the process that reduces the number of healthy cells in the body. The most striking factor in the aging process is the body's loss of reserve due to the decreasing number of cells in each organ. For example, fasting blood glucose (blood sugar) levels remain fairly constant throughout life, but the glucose-tolerance measurement shows a loss of response in aging. Glucose tolerance measures the body's ability to respond to the stress of the glucose load used to challenge the system in the test. The same diminishment holds true for the recovery mechanisms of other systems. Simply stated, aging is the body's loss of ability to respond to a challenge to its status quo (homeostasis). The mass of healthy active cells in each organ declines as a person ages, thus the organ's function is diminished.

Now the question becomes, what causes this loss of reserve? Free-radical reactions result in the body's loss of active cells. The cumulative effect of billions of cellular free-radical reactions is the loss of cells. This happens in several ways.

1. Free-radical damage to the cell membranes can impair the cell's ability to transport nutrients into the cell, and the cell dies without replacing itself.

2. Free-radical damage to cell membranes can impair the cell's ability to transport waste products out of the cell, thus the cell can become strangled by its own waste. The result is that the cell can die without replacing itself.

3. Free radicals can damage the cell's DNA so that instead of the cell being replaced by another healthy daughter cell, it is replaced with a mutant that doesn't function correctly.

4. Free radicals can damage the lysosomal sac and release deadly lysosomes, which are enzymes that destroy other cell components. This leaves the cell devoid of working parts; the cell becomes a clinker, and the body becomes one cell older.

5. Free radicals can fuse proteins together in such a fashion that the proteins do not function properly. This can damage a cell so that it does not perform and does not reproduce a healthy replacement.

6. Free-radical reactions form byproducts such as the age pigment lipofuscin or advanced glycosylated end products. These residues accumulate over time and interfere with cell function.

The result of many of the free-radical reactions is that the number of active cells in the body decreases. This is analogous to the light bulbs on an old theater marquee that burn out one by one. For a while, the message can still be read, but as the number of burned-out bulbs increases, eventually the message is indiscernible. In the body, the cells in each organ decline but the organ still functions until a point.

Since free radicals are involved in the aging process, and Pycnogenol destroys free radicals, it has an aging-retarding effect. There is one study showing that Pycnogenol extended the life span of a common laboratory species, but there is more to aging than life span. The goal is to increase the quality of life as well as the length of life. We want to add more years to our lives, but we also want to add more life to our years. Slowing the aging process is all about living better and longer.

Membrane Fluidity

As mentioned above, one of the most damaging aspects of free radicals is their effect on cell membranes. When cell membranes stiffen, the entire cell is affected and countless biochemical reactions are compromised. Pycnogenol has been shown to maintain cell membrane fluidity and thus help maintain cell function.

A 2004 study by Slovakian and Polish biochemists, published in the journal *General Physiology and Biophysics,* confirmed earlier reports that Pycnogenol improves membrane fluidity in a concentration-dependent manner.

Age-Related Diseases and Disorders

Specific age-related conditions, such as Alzheimer's disease, heart disease, arthritis, and many, many others will be discussed in subsequent chapters.

In addition to the many health benefits of Pycnogenol, there are important "vanity" benefits as well. Pycnogenol is often called the "skin vitamin" or the "oral cosmetic" because it rebuilds skin tissues, making skin more flexible and smoother and thus younger looking. It can't undo deep wrinkles or repair permanent sun damage, but it can make skin healthier. This will be discussed in Chapter 5.

Pycnogenol can help improve the *quality* of life in many ways, as well as help reduce the risk of killer diseases and help us live *better* and longer. The "quality of life" aspects will be addressed in several chapters including Chapter 9 on living life to the fullest and Chapter 10 on sexual function.

CHAPTER 4

PROTECTING THE HEART AND IMPROVING CIRCULATION

The bad news is that heart disease is a multi-faceted disease with multiple causes, yet nearly everyone focuses on cholesterol alone. In fact, in 2003, British researchers suggested that we don't need cholesterol pills as much as we need a "polypill" to address *all* the causes of heart disease. The good news is that Pycnogenol is protective against essentially all of these causes and basically is that "polypill," according to noted researcher Dr. Ronald Watson of the University of Arizona at Tucson.

Dr. Watson wrote in the journal *Evidence-Based Integrative Medicine* that there is a high probability for positive results in cardiovascular risk prevention with Pycnogenol. In his article, Dr. Watson cites some of the important heart-healthy benefits of Pycnogenol: lowering the "bad" cholesterol (LDL), raising the "good" cholesterol (HDL), reducing the "very bad" oxidized LDL cholesterol, reducing inflammation, reducing platelet aggregation, moderating high blood pressure, improving artery flexibility, and improving microcirculation.

There are several forms of heart disease, thus there are several causes. Most people think of a heart attack as the end result of heart disease, and most people associate cholesterol with heart disease. However, this isn't always the case. In this chapter, we explore the causes of heart disease and other circulatory disorders and discuss the cardiovascular benefits of Pycnogenol.

Heart Attack and Heart Disease: An Overview

When a blood clot shuts off the flow of blood in a coronary artery, the region of the heart fed by the artery is starved of oxygen and nutrients. The result is the death of these cells, which is called an infarct. This is the classic heart attack, called an acute myocardial (heart) infarction, called AMI for short.

Atherosclerosis (narrowed arteries) does not by itself cause heart attacks. Thrombosis (blood clot) and vasoconstriction (constriction and/or spasm of an artery) are the events that usually precipitate a heart attack.

Atherosclerosis
A medical term for narrowed arteries.

Narrowed arteries put the squeeze on blood platelet cells and damage them. Platelet cells are the cells that clump and clot in the blood. If you have a cut, they clot and keep you from bleeding to death. But in blood vessels, platelet aggregation leads to clots that interrupt the flow of blood. Clots can lodge in the narrowed arteries of the heart (coronary arteries), completely shutting off the flow of blood through that artery. When this happens, doctors call it a coronary thrombosis—a blood clot in a coronary artery. Hence, the expression that someone is "having a coronary."

Certain factors can cause platelets to change their shape. When a platelet changes from its normal shape, it is said to be "activated." Normally, they are activated with the intention of stopping bleeding. However, platelets can be activated even when there is no bleeding, and this is not good. If they are activated, they still tend to aggregate or clump together and initiate an undesirable blood clot that can block blood flow through the vessel and result in a heart attack or stroke.

Blood platelets
Small, disc-shaped, colorless blood cells. They are smaller than red blood cells and there are about 150,000 to 300,000 platelets per cubic centimeter of blood.

Vasoconstriction causes reduced blood flow to the heart by constricting the diameter of the artery. It can even completely shut off an artery and stop all blood flow.

High blood pressure (hypertension) affects arteries. It is a risk factor in various forms of heart disease.

Another common form of heart disease is congestive heart failure, in which the heart is too weak to pump blood efficiently. Usually, the heart enlarges as it tries to compensate for the reduced output.

Cholesterol, Lipoproteins, and Heart Disease

The process of forming so-called cholesterol deposits is very complicated, but it's important to remember that free radicals are involved and that Pycnogenol, as an antioxidant, is protective.

I have referred to the so-called bad cholesterol as LDL cholesterol, or simply LDL, and the good cholesterol as HDL cholesterol, or simply HDL. Now it's time to explore them further.

Cholesterol is needed by nearly every cell in the body. It is more efficient for the liver to make cholesterol and deliver it to the cells than for each cell to manufacture its own cholesterol. Cholesterol is not soluble in blood, so it is packaged by the liver in particles called lipoproteins, which are compatible with both cholesterol and blood. Two important lipoproteins are low-density lipoproteins (LDL) and high-density lipoproteins (HDL). The cholesterol carried by LDL is brought to the cells from the liver. This type of cholesterol is considered "bad" because it is thought to lead to cholesterol deposits. However, it becomes "bad" only after it is oxidized and becomes "oxidized LDL." The cholesterol carried by HDL is brought away from cells and back to the liver. Since it is removing cholesterol from the cells and deposits, it is considered "good."

There is good news for those who wish to lower

their LDL cholesterol and raise their good cholesterol. One clinical study at the University of Texas, Dallas, in 2002 showed that taking 150 milligrams of Pycnogenol a day significantly reduces LDL (bad) cholesterol, while it increases HDL (good) cholesterol. In the study, healthy volunteers had their blood LDL and HDL cholesterol measured before, during, and after supplementation. During Pycnogenol supplementation, there was a statistically significant drop in LDL cholesterol levels from an average of 104 to 96 milligrams per deciliter in just three weeks. When supplementation was discontinued, their LDL cholesterol values returned to their pre-supplementation levels.

In a second clinical study in the same year in Europe, conducted over three months with volunteers receiving 120 milligrams of Pycnogenol per day, showed an average 20 percent reduction in LDL cholesterol, while the "good" HDL cholesterol increased by an average of 15 percent. Again, when Pycnogenol was discontinued, cholesterol values returned to pre-supplementation levels.

Oxidized LDL

Cholesterol deposits form only when LDL becomes damaged by oxidation—that is, by free radicals. It's then called "oxidized LDL." Oxidized LDL can infiltrate the artery wall and initiate a series of events that trap the cholesterol-containing oxidized LDL inside the blood vessel wall. White blood cells, sensing that something is wrong, are attracted to the site and swell, forming what are called "foam cells" that then turn into the lesions commonly called "cholesterol deposits."

LDL is oxidized only when the amount of antioxidants is insufficient to protect the LDL against oxidation. Studies by Dr. A. Nelson and colleagues in 1998 showed that Pycnogenol directly protects LDL. However, Pycnogenol can also indirectly protect LDL. The prime antioxidant that protects LDL is vitamin E. Pycnogenol can recycle vitamin C, which, in turn, can recycle vitamin E.

Pycnogenol can also destroy the free radicals before they reach LDL to cause damage. The tendency to form oxidized LDL, and hence the cholesterol deposits (atherosclerosis), is dependent on two factors: the amount of LDL and the balance between antioxidants and free radicals. Both are important, but the antioxidant/free-radical balance is the more important of the two.

Blood Platelets and Heart Disease

Cholesterol deposits by themselves don't cause a heart attack, but they can cause angina. The cholesterol deposits are a major contributing factor to forming the blood clots that cause heart attacks. As long as the blood can squeeze by the narrowing caused by the cholesterol deposits in good volume, the heart will receive sufficient oxygen and nutrients to keep the heart tissue alive. When the blockage is severe enough to reduce the blood flow so that the heart does not receive adequate oxygen, then the pain of angina results. When blood clots form in the narrowed passage, blood flow is cut off and the area of the heart

Angina
The pain experienced in the heart when there is not enough blood reaching all parts of the heart during activity.

fed by that artery dies, resulting in a heart attack. A critical factor, then, is to maintain the proper "slipperiness" of the blood cells and prevent blood clots from forming in the coronary arteries.

Pycnogenol has a protective anti-aggregation (anticlotting) effect on blood platelets. It is particularly effective against the damage to platelets from stress and smoking.

The platelet aggregation (clumping) cycle begins when the body experiences stress, whether it's from daily activities, smoking, or even exercising. When stress results, large amounts of adrenaline are released. Adrenaline, a stress hormone, causes platelets to aggregate, narrowing arteries and restricting blood supply, and this can lead to a heart attack or stroke. Pycnogenol may benefit the entire cardiovascular system by serving as a natural shield against excessive platelet aggregation brought on by smoking and stress. Here's a completely natural substance with remarkable activity, producing effects within minutes. It may have enormous health implications for an aging population.

Several studies by Dr. Ronald Watson's research group at the University of Arizona found that Pycnogenol rapidly, within two hours, prevented platelet aggregation due to smoking. The effects of one large dose of Pycnogenol, 200 milligrams, slowed aggregation for six days. Pycnogenol, therefore, has a powerful, persistent effect of lowering adverse platelet aggregation. It is interesting to note that normal platelet clumping needed to slow bleeding was not affected. However, aspirin actually increased bleeding, an adverse side effect not found during use of Pycnogenol.

A single, smaller dose of Pycnogenol was as effective as a five times larger amount of aspirin. This is good news for the substantial portion of the population that cannot tolerate long-term aspirin use with its side effects. Studies are now underway to assess the long-term effects of Pycnogenol supplementation in nonsmokers and smokers.

While aspirin is currently recommended by cardiologists to prevent platelet aggregation, this research suggests that Pycnogenol is efficacious and safer. Of course, this is not only important in terms of heart disease, but also for preventing strokes. If platelet aggregation causes clumping and narrowing in an artery that feeds a region of the brain, a stroke is the likely result.

Another study conducted by Dr. Watson's group along with Dr. Peter Rohdewald's research team in Germany showed that Pycnogenol blocks the effect of the stress hormone adrenaline on blood platelets, thereby reducing the platelets' tendency to clump together to form blood clots. Pycnogenol is particularly effective against increased platelet aggregation caused by smoking.

Dr. Watson's research was published in *Cardiovascular Reviews Reports* in 1999 and was entitled "Reduction of Cardiovascular Disease Risk Factors by French Maritime Pine Bark Extract." A joint article by Drs. Watson, Rohdewald, and their colleagues was published in *Thrombosis Research* in 1999 as "Inhibition of Smoking-Induced Platelet Aggregation by Aspirin and Pycnogenol."

This protective effect of Pycnogenol is achieved by supporting the production of the body's own messenger molecule nitric oxide (somewhat like a hormone). Nitric oxide is produced by cells forming the inner lining of blood vessels. It acts on blood platelets to "calm them down," to stop them being in a state of alarm and "sticky," ready to form a blood clot.

Pycnogenol inhibits platelet aggregation by inhibiting the enzymes thromboxane A2, 5-lipoxygenase, and other clotting compounds. Furthermore, this protection comes without an increased risk of prolonged bleeding times, or the side effects common to aspirin. U.S. Patent No. 5,720,956 was granted for Pycnogenol's ability to inhibit platelet aggregation.

Inflammation and Heart Disease

Many recent studies have also linked inflammation to heart disease. This inflammation, specifically of blood vessel walls, is likely related to the white blood cells that are drawn to oxidized LDL. Pycnogenol reduces inflammation.

Inflammation is a normal process, but *chronic* inflammation is not. Normally, the body should turn off its inflammatory response after getting the upper hand on an infection or after an injury heals.

But if biological "switches" malfunction, the inflammatory response doesn't turn off. It's a little like leaving a car running at high idle for hours. The engine will overheat. In a sense, chronic inflammation overheats our tissues and damages them in the process.

Inflammation promotes heart disease. Oxidized LDL cholesterol may be a key instigator, along with homocysteine. *Oxidized* LDL, but not normal LDL, attracts white blood cells, which are one of the body's defenses against foreign proteins (such as bacteria or viruses) and other things that don't belong in the body. The white blood cells swallow the oxidized LDL—they recognize that oxidized LDL is not normal—and then the white blood cells stir up an inflammatory response through a number of mechanisms.

Elevated CRP levels, a marker of inflammation, are a more accurate predictor of heart attack risk than cholesterol, LDL cholesterol, homocysteine, or triglyceride. People with elevated CRP levels are four and a half times more likely to suffer a heart attack, compared with people who have normal levels. But that is only the tip of the iceberg. More details can be found in *The Inflammation Syndrome* by Jack Challem.

Pycnogenol helps in a couple of ways. As an antioxidant, it neutralizes the free radicals released by inflammation. Dr. Benjamin Lau and his colleagues at Loma Linda University showed that it also decreases the body's production of cellular adhesion molecules (CAM), which help inflammatory cells stick to blood vessel walls.

Stress, Platelet Damage, and Heart Attack

When we are under stress, our adrenaline really flows. As previously mentioned, adrenaline activates blood platelets to be prepared to clump together and form a blood clot. Furthermore, adrenaline causes blood vessels to constrict with the consequence of higher blood pressure.

Nowadays, we live under permanent stress at work, driving through traffic jams back home, and never having enough time for everything. This causes permanent constriction of blood vessels as well as continuously sticky platelets.

In consequence, the diameter of the blood vessel is reduced, leaving less space for the blood to flow. An atherosclerotic plaque may further reduce the space for blood flow. If then some platelets suddenly stick together and form a clot, the vessel may become completely clogged, causing the surrounding tissue to be deprived of nutrients and oxygen. This is how heart infarction and stroke develop.

Pycnogenol can't make the cause of your stress go away. However, it can improve the nitric oxide levels produced by cells lining the arteries. The nitric oxide instructs muscles surrounding the blood vessels to relax. At the same time, nitric oxide also tells platelets to return back to their normal "non-sticky" condition, they no longer need to be "alarmed." Thus, Pycnogenol helps the body's own mechanism to counteract the activity of the stress hormone adrenaline. Pycnogenol helps keep your blood slippery (as an anticoagulant) to reduce the chance of heart attack and stroke.

Furthermore, Pycnogenol decreases the level of thromboxane in smokers to the normal level for nonsmokers. This is an important benefit because thromboxane is a vasoconstrictor, meaning it constricts blood vessels, thereby reducing blood flow and increasing blood pressure.

Pycnogenol Protects the Lining of the Arteries

Tearing in the lining of arteries is another way in which cholesterol deposits can form. Damage to the endothelium, or lining, of the heart and arteries contributes to the risk of heart disease. This damage can cause clots to form and allow cholesterol carriers to enter the artery walls. Researchers at Loma Linda University, California, studied the protective effect of Pycnogenol using arterial endothelial cells. They found that Pycnogenol reduced the damage to endothelial cells caused by free radicals and other noxious elements. They had earlier noted that Pycnogenol increased production of other antioxidants in the cells.

The Importance of Nitric Oxide

Pycnogenol's mild hypotensive (blood-pressure-lowering) action helps maintain normal blood pressure. Blood pressure is strongly influenced by blood levels of nitric oxide, a compound that controls the relaxation of blood vessels and inhibits the angiotensin I converting enzyme (ACE), which raises blood pressure. Pycnogenol maintains adequate nitric oxide levels, controlling vasorelaxation and inhibiting ACE.

Pycnogenol helps the body to produce nitric oxide more efficiently, which makes blood platelets less sticky and dilates constricted arteries. This results in improved blood flow, and high blood pressure is counteracted.

Nitric oxide (NO) plays two very different roles in the body, a good role as well as a bad one. It is produced by cells of blood vessel walls in small quantities. As mentioned before, it is needed to cause muscles surrounding arteries to relax and keep blood platelets slippery. This is the body's own mechanism for normalizing blood flow and blood pressure.

In contrast, immune cells can produce several times more NO than that produced by blood vessel walls. In these high amounts, NO is toxic. Immune cells produce excess NO during inflammation to extinguish invading microorganisms in the case of infection. When inflammatory conditions are not accompanied by infection, the excess amounts of NO harm the body's own cells.

Pycnogenol was shown by Dr. Lester Packer of the University of California, Berkeley, to inhibit *excess* production of NO by immune cells. This is part of the anti-inflammatory action of Pycnogenol.

For healthy circulation, it is important for the cells of blood vessel walls to maintain continuous production of nitric oxide. However, many chronic inflammatory conditions cause a great deal of damage. Because immune cells produce so much NO, they cause oxidative stress and ultimately destroy the body's own cells. Immune cells perceive the situation as if it were an infection. This calls for an increase in the number and aggressiveness of immune cells. This vicious circle explains why many inflammatory disorders persist for so long. Pycnogenol, an anti-inflammatory, can help interrupt the sinister process.

Nitric oxide plays a role in many biochemical functions. It improves our memory and attention. It enhances blood flow and thereby increases kidney, lung, and liver perfusion. It preserves the functioning of the cardiovascular system. And it is responsible for the male erection.

In terms of heart disease, readers may be familiar with the fact that during angina attacks, patients find relief by taking nitroglycerin pills. These pills release nitric oxide, which relaxes the coronary arteries and allows more blood to flow into the heart.

The arteries' inner lining, called the endothelium, produces nitric oxide, which helps regulate blood flow. In addition, the nitric oxide produced in the artery lining also increases the production of a chemical messenger called cyclic-GMP (guanosine monophosphate), which is needed to keep blood platelets slippery and not prone to clumping or aggregation. Pycnogenol stimulates the enzyme nitric oxide synthase (NOS) to produce nitric oxide in the artery linings from the amino acid arginine.

Some nitric oxide is always needed, but too much can kill cells. Pycnogenol helps keep nitric oxide levels in the body at optimal levels. It helps the body produce adequate levels of nitric oxide for necessary functions, while reducing the levels of nitric oxide where it does harm.

Dr. David Fitzpatrick of the University of South Florida conducted tests to determine the effect of Pycnogenol on portions of the aorta (the main artery from the heart). He found that it improved the production of nitric oxide in the endothelium, which in turn had a relaxing effect on the aorta in a dose-dependent manner. The results were published in 1998 in the *Journal of Cardiovascular Pharmacology*.

Hypertension

Several factors, including tobacco smoking, stress, obesity, diabetes, and aging, can upset the balance between the constriction and relaxation of the blood vessels. There is increasing evidence that Pycnogenol improves this balance. As a consequence, blood can flow more easily, which results in more normal blood pressure. There are quite a few hormones and vascular mediators involved in constriction and relaxation, respectively. Dr. Ronald Watson has shown that Pycnogenol reduces production of thromboxane, a hormone-like substance that causes constriction of blood vessels. Furthermore, as mentioned earlier, Pycnogenol stimulates production of nitric oxide. This substance is produced by cells lining the blood vessel wall. Nitric oxide instructs the muscles surrounding blood vessels to relax and stop constricting. Thus, Pycnogenol supports the body's own mechanisms for better circulation.

A clinical study undertaken by Dr. Watson demonstrates Pycnogenol's profound antihypertensive action. Dr. Watson had previously shown that Pycnogenol significantly reduces high blood pressure in people who don't yet take antihypertensive medication. The new study has been carried out with hypertensive individuals who take prescribed medication containing nifedipine (a so-called calcium blocker) as the active principle. Pycnogenol was able to significantly reduce their prescribed medication without increasing their blood pressure. This positive effect did not occur in a control group receiving dummy tablets (placebo).

As Dr. Watson remarked, "We investigated mild hypertension, that not needing treatment with a pharmaceutical drug. These folks were at high risk for progressing to clinical hypertension, if therapy of exercise and diet did not lower the hypertension. Pycnogenol significantly lowered the mild hypertension down to normal blood pressure. We conclude that Pycnogenol's ability to properly dilate arteries and arterioles is responsible for the blood pressure normalizing effect." (Hosseini, S., et al. A randomized, double-blind, placebo-controlled, prospective 16-week crossover study to determine the role of Pycnogenol in modifying blood pressure in mildly hypertensive patients. *Nutrition Research* (2001) 21: 1251–260.)

Pycnogenol does have a mild hypotensive (blood-pressure-lowering) effect that helps prevent high blood pressure. This effect is important, but it does not make Pycnogenol an antihypertensive drug. There are two known reasons for Pycnogenol's hypotensive action. One mechanism involves the optimization of nitric oxide production in the blood vessels. Several researchers, including Dr. David Fitzpatrick of the University of South Florida and Dr. Lester Packer of the University of California, Berkeley, have conducted research on Pycnogenol and nitric oxide and discovered that Pycnogenol balances nitric oxide levels in the artery linings, facilitating blood flow.

Pycnogenol also has a beneficial effect on blood

pressure by blocking the action of angiotensin I converting enzyme (ACE) that causes high blood pressure. In this way, Pycnogenol is similar to, but much safer than, common prescription drugs called ACE inhibitors. ACE interferes with bradykinin, a compound that helps keep peripheral blood vessels properly dilated. Blocking this action leads to a normalization of blood pressure without the danger of driving blood pressure too low. It allows the bradykinin to act as it should, unencumbered by ACE.

Dr. Miklos Gabor and his colleagues at the Albert Szent-Györgyi Medical University in Szeged, Hungary, along with Dr. Peter Rohdewald of the University of Munster, Germany, found that Pycnogenol has a dose-dependent action in blocking ACE from raising blood pressure. Based on their study, published in 1996 in *Pharmaceutical and Pharmacological Letters,* the researchers described the hypotensive effect of Pycnogenol as "moderate." Thus, people with normal or low blood pressure will not be affected, whereas those with high blood pressure due to too much ACE will benefit. A clinical study published by Dr. Ronald Watson and colleagues at the University of Arizona in 2001 also examined this possibility.

They found a significant decrease in systolic blood pressure during Pycnogenol supplementation. Also, serum thromboxane concentration was significantly decreased during Pycnogenol supplementation. The scientists concluded, "Our data suggest that supplementation with Pycnogenol is effective in decreasing systolic blood pressure in hypertensive patients." (Araghi-Nicknam et al., Pine bark extract reduces platelet agregation. *Integrative Medicine* [1999] 2: 73–77.)

Blood Circulation

Pycnogenol helps maintain good circulation in several ways. We have already discussed how Pycnogenol improves blood flow via its effect on nitric oxide. Another way is that Pycnogenol protects the endothelial cells that line the heart and blood vessels against free radicals.

Pycnogenol also facilitates the production of "ground substance," an intercellular cement that can fill much of the space between cells in the blood vessels and control the amount of fluid and compounds that slip through. This also gives the blood vessels strength.

Pycnogenol improves blood circulation in elderly people. It does this through its antithrombotic mechanism and by causing vasodilatation through optimal production of nitric oxide from endothelium, as explained earlier.

Another way in which Pycnogenol improves circulation is by maintaining the proper flexibility of the membranes of red blood cells so that they can easily squeeze through smaller blood vessels. Several studies have shown that Pycnogenol improves membrane flexibility in red blood cells in a concentration-dependent manner—that is, the more Pycnogenol there is, the less stiff the blood cells are.

Venous Health

In addition to offering protection against many diseases, Pycnogenol also helps guard the body against venous insufficiency, varicose veins, and bruises and helps reduce the severity of minor injuries. This protection is due to the bioflavonoids in Pycnogenol rather than a general antioxidant effect.

Venous insufficiency is characterized by the feeling of heavy and swollen legs and ankles. It is particularly common in women who sit or stand in one position for prolonged periods, and in those who do not exercise. The collagen structure of veins is weakened, allowing gravity to pull plasma into the tissues of the legs and feet. Ultimately, this condition can lead to static edema and ulceration.

Pycnogenol has been shown to improve venous

health, help repair some varicose veins, and reduce the occurrence of new varicose veins. Fifteen clinical studies in venous disorders have been conducted with Pycnogenol since the 1970s. They have looked at the effect of Pycnogenol on chronic venous insufficiency, varicose veins, thrombophlebitis, post-thrombotic syndrome, and venous stasis edema. These studies have been reviewed by Dr. Om Gulati in the *European Bulletin of Drug Research* (see Selected References). Pycnogenol supplementation resulted in 89 percent of the subjects becoming free of edema, 85 percent free of swelling, 83 percent free from the feeling of "heavy" legs, and 77 percent free of nightly cramps. Sixty-nine percent of those with leg pain became pain-free.

One of the earliest discoveries about Pycnogenol was its ability to strengthen capillaries, the body's tiniest blood vessels. Early research focused on the role of Pycnogenol as either an independent factor or a cofactor with vitamin C in the maintenance of capillary health. Dr. Miklos Gabor of Albert Szent-Györgyi Medical University in Hungary conducted many studies over the years that demonstrate that Pycnogenol improves capillary permeability and decreases capillary leakage and microbleeding. The ability to bind collagen is the reason why Pycnogenol can strengthen and properly "seal" brittle vessels.

Capillaries are not designed to be completely sealed against leakage. These blood vessels are the interface between the blood stream and oxygen, nutrients, and waste products. Capillaries must be permeable enough to allow fluids to seep out, mix with the fluid that surrounds all of the cells, and then reenter. If the capillaries are too permeable, however, too much fluid and protein seep out, resulting in edema (swelling). Red blood cells may even seep out, causing bruising and red spots (petechiae) or even hematomas.

Dr. Gabor and his colleagues found that Pycnogenol improved capillary strength within two hours and maintained strength for longer than eight hours. They have described their findings in the journal *Phlebologie* (1993).

Dr. F. Feine-Haake studied the benefit of Pycnogenol on 100 persons with varicose veins and other symptoms of chronic venous insufficiency. They were given 30 milligrams of Pycnogenol three times a day (a total of 90 milligrams). Eighty percent showed a clear improvement, and 90 percent found that their nocturnal leg cramps also disappeared.

Pycnogenol helps keep all of the blood vessels healthy and reduces edema, which contributes to the development of varicose veins. In double-blind, placebo-controlled studies it has been shown that Pycnogenol greatly improves symptoms of chronic venous insufficiency.

Clinical studies and laboratory animal studies show that Pycnogenol reduces water retention and swelling in the legs due to edema. It does this by strengthening capillaries and preventing leakage of fluids.

Pycnogenol helps maintain capillary strength and proper capillary permeability, thus guarding against spontaneous bruising. A bruise is pooled blood beneath the surface of the skin. If the capillaries leak too much, fluid and proteins can leak through the capillaries into the neighboring spaces between cells, thereby altering the normal osmotic pressure. Eventually, even red blood cells can leak through and spontaneously cause a bruise without a direct injury to the capillaries. Pycnogenol restores proper permeability and reduces the incidence of spontaneous bruising. With stronger capillaries, it will take a more forceful injury to damage the veins and capillaries enough to allow microbleeding into the tissues.

Economy-Class Syndrome

The name of this condition may be a little misleading, as long-haul flights affect all passengers to a marked degree. Of course, there are more economy-class passengers and they have less room to move about, which does compound the problem. Long-haul air flights lead to passenger dehydration due to the low-humidity of the cabin and insufficient fluid intake. Alcohol only adds to the problem, causing a further thickening of the blood. Dehydration causes the blood to thicken and turn to "sludge." Blood flow slows by as much as two-thirds, allowing blood platelets to interact more closely. This increases platelet aggregation and the risk of deep vein thrombosis. Inactivity and sitting for long periods without moving the legs much adds to the problem.

Observational studies have suggested that on long-haul flights up to 10 percent of passengers may be affected, although the majority of thromboses that occur during travel remain symptom-free, as the developed clot spontaneously dissolves before it may affect blood flow. However, thrombosis may be fatal when the blood clot is dislodged and blocks the branches of arteries in the lungs (pulmonary embolism).

A double-blind, placebo-controlled study, published in the October 2004 issue of *Clinical Applied Thrombosis/Hemostasis*, demonstrated Pycnogenol's protective effect during long-haul flights. The trial included 198 subjects who either supplemented with Pycnogenol or a placebo. They took 200 milligrams two to three hours prior to a long-haul flight, 200 milligrams six hours later in mid-flight, and 100 milligrams the day after flying. The flights used in the test lasted an average of eight hours and fifteen minutes. Researchers concluded that Pycnogenol treatment was effective in protecting against thrombotic events (DVT) and superficial vein thrombosis (SVT) in moderate- to high-risk subjects during long-haul flights as compared to the placebo group that produced five thrombotic events.

Dr. Peter Rohdewald of the study group concluded, "Travel-related DVT and SVT are preventable conditions. Pycnogenol is one of the most powerful natural antioxidants available today and has the ability to control the permeability of capillary walls, preventing edema, inhibiting platelet aggregation and ultimately reducing thrombotic events."

Personally, I wouldn't think of getting on a plane without taking extra Pycnogenol. If my flight is longer than four hours, I take even more Pycnogenol at the four-hour mark. I have seen too many people develop clots on flights, and more who have embolisms lodge in their lungs a day or two after their flight as the clot dislodges from the leg vein and travels through the body.

The so-called economy-class syndrome is not limited to economy-class flights. This condition has been blamed for at least thirty deaths in three years at just one hospital in London, England. Sitting still in airplane seats encourages blood to pool in the ankles. The edge of the seat tends to reduce the return flow of blood through the leg veins. One result is that the ankles can swell, but a worse result is that a blood clot can form in the deep veins of the legs and then travel as an embolism to a coronary artery and cause a heart attack, or to the brain and cause a stroke. In addition, the reduced oxygen levels and increased radiation levels during high-altitude flights increases the need for the powerful antioxidant protection of Pycnogenol.

When you are trapped in a plane at high altitude, breathing germs from your neighbors for hours at a time, getting zapped by cosmic radiation, breathing low levels of oxygen, you definitely would benefit from extra Pycnogenol. The first thing you will notice is that your shoes fit upon arrival. Airlines should be required to distribute Pycnogenol supplements in-flight just like they used to pass out chewing gum to help ease ear problems during changes in cabin pressure.

Remaining in a sitting position for long periods of time during long-haul flights also increases the risk of blood platelets forming a clot. When the blood clot travels to an artery in the lung, it may get stuck there and block blood flow. This pulmonary embolism often has a fatal outcome. As previously mentioned, Pycnogenol has shown in several studies to keep blood platelets in the bloodstream slippery. This helps to prevent the much-feared pulmonary embolism.

A much more common problem during long-haul flights, though surely not life-threatening, is the phenomenon of lower legs and feet becoming swollen. This occurs because venous blood pressure increases in the lower limbs, causing small capillaries to leak plasma into the surrounding tissue. Pycnogenol strengthens and seals brittle blood capillaries and has been shown in several clinical studies to counteract swelling in the feet and lower legs. However, the phenomenon most people experience when they take Pycnogenol on long-haul flights is that their shoes fit when they arrive at their destination!

CHAPTER 5

SKIN CARE
WITH PYCNOGENOL

S kin is more than beauty—it is a vital organ that protects us from the environment, maintains hydration and body temperature, and is part of the immune system. Pycnogenol has been called "the skin vitamin" by many users. However, as explained earlier, Pycnogenol is not a vitamin, but a nutritional supplement. It has also been popularly called "the oral cosmetic" because it gives skin a more vibrant glow. Pycnogenol renews skin by rebuilding tissue, making skin more flexible, smoother, healthier, and younger looking. Pycnogenol can't undo deep wrinkles or repair the permanent sun damage of actinic keratosis, but it can make skin healthier, livelier, tighter, firmer, more elastic, smoother, and with fewer fine lines and less discoloration. Supplementation with Pycnogenol shows visible results, as proven in clinical studies.

Also, topical application of Pycnogenol works well. It directly nourishes the skin and is nonirritating. An aqueous solution containing 5 percent Pycnogenol can be absorbed by the skin in four to six hours.

Pycnogenol improves skin by its action with skin proteins and by improving the microcirculation that hydrates, oxygenates, and nourishes the skin. This improved microcirculation also clears toxins from the skin more quickly. As explained at the beginning of this book, Pycnogenol's first commercial uses were based on its ability to improve the permeability of blood capillaries. Soon it was also learned that Pycnogenol improved skin by promoting and protecting the skin proteins collagen and elastin.

Pycnogenol has a specific, high affinity for collagen and elastin. Like a "magic bullet," it finds its way to these skin proteins, binds to them, and protects them against free radicals and destructive enzymes!

Studies have also shown that Pycnogenol helps produce new collagen fibers. This helps make skin smoother and more elastic. Pycnogenol gives the skin a more vibrant glow.

Skin Smoothness

In addition to its protective benefits against free radicals, which prevents skin damage, Pycnogenol binds to collagen and elastin, and protects these proteins from various enzymes that break them down. This action reduces the thinning of skin that develops with aging. Pycnogenol helps the skin rebuild its thickness and elasticity. Skin fullness and elasticity are essential for skin smoothness.

Sun Damage to Skin

As skin ages, it loses its flexibility. This is primarily due to the cumulative effect of sun exposure, which alters the skin structure and reduces the amount of skin protein produced. You can easily see this effect. When young skin is pinched and pulled up, it will spring back quickly. When older skin is similarly pinched, it returns to position very slowly. Try this on the back of the hands of people of various ages. How does your skin do?

Have you ever noticed that the skin on the back of the necks of farmers and fishermen is thick, leathery, and deeply wrinkled compared to the skin of office workers? You can also compare the apparent age of skin on different areas of your own body. We tend to think of our skin as being the same age as our chronological age, but the fact is that some cells are much newer than others.

Compare the smoothness of the skin on a sun-exposed area, such as the back of your neck, to the skin on a sun-protected area, such as your buttocks. The sun is what made the difference, by causing free radicals to fuse molecules of the skin protein collagen together.

The proteins in young skin slide freely over one another and spring back to their normal length when stretched. As time goes by and exposure to the sun accumulates, the ultraviolet energy in sunlight interacts with fats in the skin to produce free radicals. These free radicals damage proteins in the skin and can link the proteins together. These damaged proteins do not easily slide over one another and do not recoil quickly. How does Pycnogenol fit in? By neutralizing free radicals, Pycnogenol can lessen sun damage to skin.

People who are well protected by antioxidants, such as Pycnogenol, find that their skin does not "burn" as quickly in the sun. Sunburn is an inflammation caused by the free radicals that are produced by the effect of sunlight on fats in the skin. Free-radical damage can be limited by the scavenging function of antioxidants. Studies have shown that the time of exposure required for sunburn to develop can be increased with Pycnogenol, but Pycnogenol should not be your only protection from the sun. The use of sunblock, wearing a hat, and an awareness of exposure time are also important.

Pycnogenol can be used as an internal as well as an external sunscreen. In clinical studies, Dr. Peter Rohdewald of the University of Munster in Germany marked different areas of the forearm, applied different strengths of Pycnogenol to these areas, and then exposed the forearm to sunlight. Pycnogenol protected the skin in a dose-related manner, meaning that higher concentrations were better than lower concentrations. Several other researchers have extended these studies and shown that human volunteers were more resistant to UV irradiation when they had taken Pycnogenol tablets. They also discovered that Pycnogenol prevents inflammation of the UV-exposed skin.

Earlier studies had been conducted in Finland by Dr. Antii Arstila of the University of Jyvaeskylae. Dr. Arstila found that Pycnogenol reduced sun damage to skin—both induced cytotoxicity and lipid peroxidation in a manner proportional to the amount of Pycnogenol present. In the United States in 2001, Drs. Lester Packer (University of California, Berkeley) and Ronald Watson (University of Arizona, Tucson) showed that four weeks of Pycnogenol supplementation increased the time it took for skin to redden in the sun. Higher doses resulted in an even longer amount of time, almost twice as long, before skin sunburned.

Wound Healing

Pycnogenol helps heal the skin and reduces scaring. Cuts, tears, and wounds initiate an inflammatory response. An over-response of the inflammatory process or a lack of collagen production hampers healing. The length of time it takes for such wounds to heal properly increases as we age. Treating wounds topically with Pycnogenol has been shown to be more effective than the body's most powerful anti-inflammatory compound, hydrocortisone.

Pycnogenol provides a combination of actions. In addition to rebuilding skin protein, improving microcirculation, and sparing vitamin C, Pycnogenol is an anti-inflammatory and an antimicrobial.

A study published in *Phytotherapy Research* in 2004 demonstrated that Pycnogenol protects the collagen matrix and increases skin stability during healing. A topical gel containing 3 percent Pycnogenol shortened healing time by three days, while a 1 percent Pycnogenol gel reduced healing by more than a day and a half. Scar formation was less pronounced with both concentrations. The researchers concluded that Pycnogenol is a potent material for the treatment of minor injuries.

Psoriasis

Psoriasis is characterized by capillary bleeding associated with increased capillary fragility. The capillary resistance of psoriatic patients is significantly lower than that of healthy persons. According to Dr. Miklos Gabor of the Albert Szent-Györgyi Medical University in Hungary, Pycnogenol helps improve capillary resistance.

Although there are no clinical studies to verify this action, holistic physicians in Europe and in the United States have experienced good results treating psoriasis patients with Pycnogenol. Many have unexpectedly found that when Pycnogenol was given to patients for other disorders, the patients' psoriasis suddenly cleared up. A recent study by Dr. Packer has revealed how Pycnogenol can be effective against psoriasis and other skin disorders: it acts on genes encoding inflammatory molecules. Pycnogenol reduces production of these molecules, and thus turns off the inflammation.

Hyperpigmentation (Melasma, Chloasma)

Melasma (chloasma) is an overpigmentation of the skin that affects sun-exposed areas of the skin such as the face. This disorder occurs mainly in women. The cause of the condition is unknown, but it is widely believed to be related to the hormonal status of women, associated with oral contraceptives, pregnancy, and recent birth. Dr. Ni Zhigang and his colleagues at the Chinese Academy of Traditional Chinese Medicine found thirty days of treatment with 75 milligrams of Pycnogenol daily to be very effective and safe. In their study, 80 percent of patients responded very favorably, with the area and the intensity of hyperpigmentation greatly reduced.

CHAPTER 6

SYNDROME X
AND DIABETES

Syndrome X and diabetes mellitus are two disorders that are rapidly increasing in occurrence in the modern world. Both are conditions in which the body cannot properly convert food into energy, resulting from improper insulin function. In both cases, Pycnogenol can help.

Syndrome X

Syndrome X, also called the insulin-resistance syndrome or the metabolic syndrome, is the term used to define a cluster of two or more of the following traits: abdominal obesity (paunch or beer belly), high blood pressure, high cholesterol, high triglycerides, and insulin resistance. Insulin resistance—a form of glucose intolerance that prevents the body from efficiently using insulin—is the cornerstone of Syndrome X, and it leads to all of these other problems.

Syndrome X and its underlying insulin resistance are major risk factors for adult-onset diabetes and heart disease. However, it also accelerates the whole aging process and the development of degenerative diseases, going way beyond diabetes and heart disease and including cancer and Alzheimer's disease.

The cause may be a diet high in refined carbohydrates. Basically, if you are eating the typical American diet, with all of its pastas, breads, cereals, and sweets, you're on the fast track to developing insulin resistance and Syndrome X. What happens is this: large amounts of refined carbohydrates and sugar trigger a rapid increase in blood sugar levels. In response, the pancreas quickly releases large amounts of the hormone insulin, which normally moves the blood sugar into cells, where it's to be burned for energy. But the insulin receptors on cells eventually get overwhelmed by the excess insulin, and cells become insulin resistant. In other words, cells cannot properly use insulin to burn sugar. As a result, more and more of the glucose is converted to fat and stored, and some remains in the blood, leading eventually to adult-onset diabetes. More information on Syndrome X can be found in *Syndrome X: The Complete Nutritional Program to Prevent and Reverse Insulin Resistance* by Jack Challem, Burt Berkson, M.D., Ph.D., and Melissa Diane Smith.

Pycnogenol reduces the damage resulting from high blood sugar whether it be mildly high such as in Syndrome X or exceedingly high such as in diabetes. These actions of Pycnogenol will be discussed in the next section.

Diabetes

Diabetes mellitus is a disorder in which the body cannot properly convert foods into energy. The damage to the cells that leads to either type 1 (juvenile) diabetes or type 2 (adult-onset) diabetes involves free-radical reactions. Once there has been damage to the islets of Langerhans cells of the pancreas (as in type 1 diabetes) or to cellular mechanisms for utilizing insulin (as in type 2 diabetes), antioxidants cannot reverse the damage.

Diabetes itself increases the production of free radicals, which further damage the body and increase the risk of heart attack, nerve damage (diabetic neuropathy), cataract (diabetic cataract), blindness (diabetic retinopathy), and other complications. Here's where powerful antioxidant protection is especially needed—diabetics need more antioxidant protection than healthy persons. Pycnogenol is the most powerful antioxidant nutrient known at this time.

Also with diabetes, the chronically increased blood sugar level adversely affects the integrity of blood vessel walls, causing them to become both stiffer and leaky. In diabetics' eyes, blood leaks through the blood vessels (microbleeding) and spills onto the retina, causing progressive loss of vision and, ultimately, blindness.

Five clinical studies conducted in Europe involving more than 1,200 diabetics showed that Pycnogenol at 20–160 milligrams per day over six months restores capillaries to their proper permeability, thus sealing adverse leaks and greatly reducing symptoms in patients with diabetic retinopathies, maculopathies, and other visual dysfunctions. The vision (visual acuity) of treated patients not only stopped decreasing further but even improved.

Elevated blood sugar levels also increase damage to proteins. This damage can be evaluated by measuring the blood level of glycosylated protein. This measurement is of great value because it measures the effect of blood sugar over time as opposed to measuring blood sugar directly, which only indicates that value at the instant that the blood is drawn. In 2003, a study in China by Dr. Y. Zhang and colleagues determined that Pycnogenol reduces the levels of glycosylated protein in diabetics, thus showing that Pycnogenol lowers blood sugar over extended periods of time.

In 2004, two clinical studies conducted in China supported the earlier studies. The first double-blind, placebo-controlled study found that seventy-seven type 2 diabetics who continued to take their anti-diabetic medication further lowered blood sugar levels and increased cardiovascular function during supplementation with Pycnogenol.

The patients in this study took 100 milligrams of Pycnogenol for twelve weeks at the same time as a standard antidiabetic treatment. The researchers from the Guang An Men Hospital of Chinese Medical Science Research Institute in Beijing and the University of Munster in Germany concluded, "Supplementation of Pycnogenol to conventional diabetes treatment lowers blood sugar levels and improves endothelial function" (*Life Sciences* 75 (21):2505–13). The second factor the researchers cite, endothelial function, is very important. This refers to the functioning of the inner lining of the arteries. While controlling blood sugar is important, it is so because elevated levels damage the blood vessels and increases the risk of heart disease. So, the clinical measurement of improved blood vessel health—endothelial function—is of the utmost importance.

The researchers state that the distinct decrease of endothelin-1 levels together with the increase of thromboxane concentrations point to a remarkable recovery of blood vessel function during Pycnogenol supplementation. Endothelin-1 levels are elevated in type 2 diabetics and atherosclerosis patients. Supplementation with Pycnogenol shifts the balance between the vasoconstricting effect of endothelin-1 and the vasodilating effect of prostacyclin toward vasodilatation, and thus benefits patients with diabetes type 2, in addition to lowering blood sugar levels.

The researchers point out that Pycnogenol helps diabetics by reducing oxidative stress and stimulating the production of nitric oxide synthase, which enhances nitric oxide production. This, in turn, improves vasodilatation and inhibits endothelin-1 production and undesirable blood platelet aggregation.

The second 2004 clinical study, published in *Diabetes Care* in March 2004, was an open, controlled, dose-finding study. Thirty type-2 diabetics between the ages of twenty-eight and sixty-four were given 50, 100, 200, and 300 milligrams of Pycnogenol in succession, with increases every three weeks. The study found that Pycnogenol lowered blood sugar in a dose-dependent manner

The inhibition of platelet aggregation by Pycnogenol is especially important to type 2 diabetics. Type 2 diabetics have been shown to have increased blood platelet aggregation and an especially high risk of blood clots, which can lead to coronary thrombosis and result in heart attacks. Eighty percent of type 2 diabetics die from such events.

A major concern of diabetics is diabetic retinopathy. When the capillaries feeding the retina leak, vision is impaired; eventually, this can lead to blindness. Elevated blood sugar also damages the capillaries and makes them brittle and swollen. Diabetic retinopathy is the leading cause of blindness in persons under the age of sixty in industrialized countries. Twenty years after the onset of diabetes, over 90 percent of type 1 diabetics and over 60 percent of type 2 diabetics develop diabetic retinopathy.

Several studies have shown that Pycnogenol is effective in halting the progression of retinopathy. Some studies have shown that Pycnogenol actually improves retinal health. For example, Professors E. Balestrazzi and L. Spadea of the University of Aquila, Italy, demonstrated Pycnogenol benefits in diabetic retinopathy. They treated diabetic retinopathy patients for two months with either a placebo or 150 milligrams of Pycnogenol per day. Visual acuity worsened in the patients receiving the placebo, as was expected, but acuity improved in those receiving Pycnogenol. This was due to Pycnogenol's ability to stop the microbleeding in the retina.

A 2002 multicenter clinical study under the direction of Drs. Frank Schonlau and Peter Rohdewald also showed that Pycnogenol stopped retinal degeneration and improved visual acuity. In this study, 1,169 patients with diabetic retinopathy were treated with daily dosages of 40 to 160 milligrams of Pycnogenol per day for six months. The trend toward improved vision was observable after three months, and further improvement continued throughout the remainder of the study.

Another condition of great concern to diabetics is diabetic cataract. Since diabetics produce more free radicals, and free radicals can cause cataracts, diabetics have a greater incidence of this eye condition. Pycnogenol's effect on cataracts will be discussed in Chapter 9.

CHAPTER 7

ALLERGIES AND ASTHMA

Pycnogenol's ability to help reduce the risk of killer diseases involving free radicals, such as cancer and heart disease, is a relatively new discovery. Decades before Pycnogenol's antioxidant roles were known, it was successfully used in Europe to control hay fever. It has also been known for decades that Pycnogenol fights inflammation, although the reason wasn't clear until recently.

Allergies

Allergies are hypersensitive reactions that occur when the body comes in contact with harmless substances that it perceives as harmful. Substances that cause these reactions are termed allergens. When a hypersensitive person comes into contact with an allergen, the body releases histamine in an attempt to fight off the allergen. This release of histamine triggers the symptoms so common to allergies—inflammation, sneezing, runny nose, and itchy eyes.

Bioflavonoids block histamine release in *in vitro* studies. Professor Sharma from the Department of Pharmacology of the University of Dublin in Ireland has shown that Pycnogenol inhibits histamine *release* from specific body cells (mast cells). This action is made possible by Pycnogenol's free-radical scavenging property. These findings were presented during the British Pharmacology Society meetings held in Dublin in July 2001 and were published in 2003 in *Phytotherapy Research*.

Antihistamines generally work by interfering

with histamine's *attachment* to cells after it has been released. However, it's more efficient to prevent histamine release in the first place, as Pycnogenol does, than to try to keep released histamine away from its receptors on target cells.

Bioflavonoids also appear to increase the uptake and reuptake of histamine into its storage granules, where it's out of the way and can't cause misery.

What may prove to be a third important mechanism was reported by Dr. David White of the University of Nottingham in England. Dr. White's studies suggest that Pycnogenol blocks the action of an enzyme called histidine decarboxylase, which produces histamine from the amino acid histidine.

Pycnogenol may be effective against allergies resulting from airborne allergens without producing side effects such as drowsiness and dry mucous membranes. Pycnogenol has not been tested against allergic reactions to insect bites and food allergens, and because these allergens can be potentially life-threatening, such use is not recommended at this time.

Asthma

Asthma is a condition that terrorizes sufferers as they can't seem to breathe because of difficulty in exhaling air from the lungs. They suffer episodes of "wheezy" breathlessness. Asthma is believed to be caused by inflammation of the bronchi, which causes them to swell and constrict their open passageways, thereby impeding the airways. The anti-inflammatory action of Pycnogenol helps asthmatics breathe more easily.

The mechanisms that cause asthma are similar to those of hay fever. Asthma can result from the immune system mistakenly perceiving a harmless foreign substance like pollen or animal hair as potentially dangerous. As a result, the bronchi begin to swell, causing severe breathing problems.

Often the vicious inflammation cycle that occurs causes asthmatic attacks to persist over long periods of time.

In 2001, a study by Dr. Ron Watson's research team at the University of Arizona, Tucson, showed that the anti-inflammatory activity of Pycnogenol was very helpful for people suffering from asthma. They were able to breathe more easily. The percentage of total lung volume that asthmatics could exhale within a second rose considerably after taking Pycnogenol at a dosage of 1 milligram per pound of body weight per day. Also, leukotrienes (pro-inflammatory molecules in the bloodstream) were shown to be lower after supplementation with Pycnogenol. The placebo had no effect. The study was a randomized, double-blind, placebo-controlled, cross-over design.

CHAPTER 8

ARTHRITIS
AND LUPUS

Lupus and some forms of arthritis involve immune-system dysfunction. Pycnogenol is an effective anti-inflammatory nutrient that has been show to benefit sufferers of both conditions.

Arthritis

Arthritis is a multifaceted disease, possibly having several causes. The word "arthritis" is derived from a Greek word meaning "joint" and actually means inflammation of the joint. Arthritis, like other degenerative diseases discussed in this book, is either caused by or involves free radicals in its pathology.

Arthritis is characterized by swelling, pain, localized heat, and redness. This inflammation can occur due to irritation or injury. Fluid gets trapped in the spaces between cells in the injured tissue. This fluid most often is the result of leakage from capillaries, but it can also be produced within the tissue by way of free-radical reactions. Inflammatory cells migrate into inflamed tissue and produce excessive amounts of free radicals.

Pycnogenol inhibits accumulation of inflammatory cells, and reduces the output of inflammatory substances. It helps normalize capillary permeability to prevent the leakage of fluid that causes edema (swelling). It also helps by neutralizing free radicals that promote swelling and inflammation.

When people with arthritis take Pycnogenol for other disorders, they are often surprised to find that their arthritic aches and pains improve as well. This benefit should not be all that surprising because arthritis is an inflammatory disease that involves free radicals. Reducing free radicals eases the swelling associated with inflammation and improves the arthritic condition.

A free radical called the superoxide anion is involved in the inflammation of arthritis. In studies, injections of superoxide dismutase, an antioxidant that quenches the superoxide free radical, reduced arthritic swelling and inflammation. Experiments by several investigators have shown that Pycnogenol also quenches superoxide anion free radicals (see review article by Packer et al., 1999, listed in Selected References).

Lupus

Systemic lupus erythematosus (SLE) is a multisystem autoimmune disease characterized by multiple immune dysfunction at the molecular and cellular levels. SLE is considered a chronic inflammatory disease.

Lupus can affect virtually any system in the body. It can be thought of as a "self-allergy" in which the body attacks its own cells and tissues, especially the skin, joints, blood, and kidneys, causing inflammation, pain, and possible organ damage.

Pycnogenol's anti-inflammatory action reduces the aggressiveness of the immune system toward its own body. Dr. S. Szegli and his Bucharest colleagues investigated Pycnogenol in the treatment of lupus and concluded, "Pycnogenol was useful for second line therapy to reduce the inflammatory feature of lupus." (Stefanescu et al., "Pycnogenol efficacy in the treatment of systemic lupus erythematosus patients." *Phytotherapy Research* 2001 15: 698–704.) Their study also found that lupus patients who took Pycnogenol along with their prescribed medication had lower amounts of these rebel antibodies. Pycnogenol, then, was shown to help protect the normal healthy components of the patients' bodies.

CHAPTER 9

LIVE LIFE TO THE FULLEST

It's uncanny how many people have been introduced to the benefits of nutritional supplements because they have developed eye problems. There will be many more as the "baby boomers" age. Dry eyes, glaucoma, and cataracts start to become problems in the fifty-plus years. Later on, age-related macular degeneration looms as a real danger.

The good news is that Pycnogenol has been shown to improve a wide range of health conditions that increasingly impact our lives as we age—including visual acuity, oral health, and endurance. Research on Pycnogenol's impact on mental function and Alzheimer's disease is still in its infancy, but preliminary findings are encouraging. In this chapter, we will take a look at how Pycnogenol can help us all live life to the fullest.

Visual Acuity

One recent poll listed the possibility of vision loss as the number-two fear of senior citizens, second only to the fear of cancer. Pycnogenol not only helps defend the body against cancer by hunting down free radicals, but it has also been shown to improve visual acuity and suspend the deterioration of retinal function that can lead to blindness. Much of this research stems from clinical studies of diabetic retinopathy, which we looked at in Chapter 6, but the results apply to nondiabetics as well.

A double-blind, placebo-controlled study published in *Phytotherapy* in May 2001 demonstrated that Pycnogenol improves visual acuity in patients suffering from diabetes, atherosclerosis, and other diseases. Those receiving 50 milligrams of Pycnogenol three times a day had either an improvement in visual acuity or a slower rate of loss of acuity compared to those in the control group receiving a placebo (an inert pill).

Pycnogenol helps protect the eye lens against the free radicals generated by sunlight. Pycnogenol's antioxidant power can help spare the vision-related nutrients, the carotenoids lutein and zeaxanthin, that are lacking in the diet but which protect the center of vision, the eye's macula.

In *in vitro* (test-tube) studies in Japan that looked at the ability of antioxidants to prevent damage of the very sensitive lipids of the eye retina, researchers found that Pycnogenol was the most effective supplement. They found that Pycnogenol protected retinal tissue far better than grape seed extract or vitamins C and E. Pycnogenol was 1.5 times more effective than catechin and at least 10 times more potent than grape seed extract, 40 times more potent than vitamin E, 350 times more potent than vitamin C, and 1,000 times more potent than lipoic acid. These results corroborate earlier *in vitro* studies that also found Pycnogenol to be more effective in protecting the retina than several other antioxidants.

Cataracts

Cataracts are associated with aging, but they are caused by free radicals, not time. Sunlight is the main source of free radicals that damage the eye lens. Several epidemiological studies have shown that various antioxidant nutrients reduce the incidence of cataracts. Since Pycnogenol is water soluble, it can bathe the eye with its powerful combination of antioxidants.

A study by Dr. J. R. Trevithick of the University of Western Ontario in Canada has shown that Pycnogenol helps to prevent cataract development in diabetic rats.

Oral Health

Pycnogenol has demonstrated a great number of oral health benefits. In addition to reducing periodontitis (a disease of the periodontium characterized by inflammation of the gums, resorption of the alveolar bone, and degeneration of the periodontal membrane) and general inflammation of the gums, Pycnogenol significantly reduces gum bleeding and plaque formation.

A study performed at Loma Linda University in California, using Pycnogenol in chewing gum (5 milligrams per stick), greatly outperformed sugar-free chewing gum. Dental students chewed six pieces of either Pycnogenol gum or sugar-free gum per day over a period of two weeks. Those chewing the Pycnogenol gum had more than a 50 percent reduction in gum bleeding, while those chewing the sugar-free gum had no reduction. The Pycnogenol group had significant reduction in plaque, while the sugar-free group showed a significant increase in plaque. Lead researcher, Dr. Benjamin Lau, concluded that with Pycnogenol gum, "individuals who enjoy chewing gum may reduce the need for frequent tooth brushing and, at the same time, increase the benefits of maintaining gingival health." (Kimbrough, C. et al. Pycnogenol minimized gingival bleedings and plaque. *Phytomedicine* 2002; 9: 410–413.)

Another study at the University of Barcelona in Spain found that Pycnogenol powder had an antimicrobial effect against a broad range of microorganisms, including the plaque formers *Streptococcus glucans* and *Candida albicans*. One patient who developed a *Candida* infection in his mouth after receiving radiation treatment for his neck cancer did not respond to conventional antifungal drug treatment. But after a month of chewing Pycnogenol tablets, he had no trace of *Candida.*

Pycnogenol can also be used in a mouth spray to promote oral health. A commercial mouth spray containing 2 milligrams of Pycnogenol per squirt is popular in Finland as a means of reducing swelling, inflammation, and bleeding in denture wearers. This practice improves denture fit and gum health.

Improving Memory and Mental Function

Animal learning and memory studies can provide us with a good indication of what will apply to humans. Dr. Benjamin Lau and his colleagues at Loma Linda University in California investigated memory retention and learning ability of mice. They discovered that older mice given Pycnogenol for two months almost reached the mental retention levels of young mice.

Alzheimer's Disease

It is too early to tell how Pycnogenol affects Alzheimer's disease, but laboratory studies are underway. We do know that Pycnogenol shields brain cells from the oxidative stress of free radicals. One of the characteristics of Alzheimer's disease is the accumulation of the protein beta-amyloid. Dr. R. Schubert and his colleagues at the Salk Institute of Biological Sciences in San Diego have found that Pycnogenol prevents the toxic action of that protein against brain cells in laboratory experiments.

Dr. Lester Packer and colleagues at the University of California at Berkeley have found that Pycnogenol protects brain cells from damage from excessive amounts of toxic glutamate.

Endurance

Exercise is beneficial in many ways, but few people realize that exercise increases the need for antioxidants. Sports and exercise require that we burn more calories for energy and thus we use more oxygen. When we consume more oxygen, we unfortunately create more free radicals. If we are deficient in antioxidants, the benefits of exercise are diminished by the damage from free radicals. The message here is not to reduce exercise or activity, but to be sure that you get adequate nourishment including ample antioxidants. As has been stated throughout this book, Pycnogenol is a powerful antioxidant. Added to that, it improves blood circulation.

A study supports the observation that Pycnogenol improves athletic endurance. Dr. Paul Pavlovic of the Department of Physical Education and Exercise Physiology at California State University found that in a double-blind, cross-over design clinical trial, the twenty-four persons receiving 200 milligrams of Pycnogenol daily for thirty days had an improvement in endurance of 21 percent, compared to the time they did not take Pycnogenol. Endurance was measured by parameters such as maximal oxygen consumption.

CHAPTER 10

SEXUAL FUNCTION, FERTILITY, AND MENSTRUAL DISORDERS

By now, it should be no surprise to learn that sexual function and dysfunction can be affected by free radicals. Perhaps this subject doesn't seem as important to many readers as the killer diseases, but for those suffering from infertility or other such disorders, this subject can be more important than the killer diseases.

Improved Fertility

Horse breeders swear by Pycnogenol, if that's any indication of its ability to promote fertility. Sperm is extremely vulnerable to oxidative stress because it contains large quantities of polyunsaturated fatty acids (PUFA). The high amounts of PUFA make membranes of sperm very soft and flexible. The development of sperm takes ninety days. If during that time a man lives unhealthily, is exposed to pollution, or just lives under heavy stress, the resulting oxidative stress destructs the membranes of the developing sperm.

Pycnogenol is such a powerful antioxidant that it helps prevent destruction of sperm membranes. Antioxidants in general improve sperm motility and mobility. Vitamin C, selenium, lipoic acid, and vitamin E are also useful in improving fertility.

Dr. Scott Roseff and colleagues at the West Essex Center for Advanced Reproductive Endocrinology in West Orange, New Jersey, found that 200 milligrams of Pycnogenol taken daily for ninety days increased the percentage of structurally normal sperm—that is, non-deformed sperm—by an average of 99 percent. Sperm count did not change. They suggest that this 99 percent increase in structurally normal sperm may allow couples diagnosed with certain types of infertility to forgo *in vitro* fertilization in favor of less invasive and less expensive fertility-promoting procedures. It is important to take Pycnogenol continuously over long periods of time—at least ninety days, the time necessary for sperms to get mature.

In a study in Europe, 40 percent of couples having difficulties in conceiving because of sperm quality were successful after using Pycnogenol for a year.

Menstrual Cramps and Endometriosis

Dysmenorrhea is characterized by spasmodic symptoms, such as severe lower abdominal pain, lumbago, headache, and nausea, which develop at the onset of and during menstruation and which are not attributable to other gynecological disorders (adnexitis, endometriosis, uterine myoma, adenomyosis of the uterus, and so on). The causes of dysmenorrhea include increased presence of prostaglandins in the menstrual fluid and an abrupt increase in intrauterine pressure caused by the menstrual fluid held in the uterus due to the constriction of os uteri.

Pycnogenol has been awarded a patent (U.S. Patent No. 6,372,266 granted on April 16, 2002) for its benefits in menstrual disorders, including dysmenorrhea and endometriosis. In Japanese studies, Pycnogenol proved to be helpful in cases in which women suffered from severe menstrual pain. Pycnogenol was particularly effective against menstrual cramping pain.

Pycnogenol itself is not a painkiller per se. It doesn't treat the symptom of pain but rather the cause of the pain. Some of Pycnogenol's constituents prevent the uterine muscle from causing cramps. Furthermore, Pycnogenol helps the blood vessels ruptured during menstruation to recover more easily.

In the Japanese study cited above, some women were diagnosed with endometriosis. In endometriosis, the cells normally lining the uterus—those cells that are shed during menstruation—are growing elsewhere in the abdominal cavity. During menstruation, these cells are not shed like the ones in the uterus. Instead, they become inflamed, and this is extremely painful, even incapacitating. The Japanese researchers showed that the anti-inflammatory activity of Pycnogenol helps in cases of endometriosis.

In a study by Drs. Takafumi Kohama and Nobutaka Suzuki of the School of Medicine at Kanazawa University, Japan, Pycnogenol was given to women as a daily dose of 30–60 milligrams daily for four weeks, beginning two weeks before their period. (It is important to start taking Pycnogenol at least one week before the menstrual period starts.) A decrease or complete disappearance of pain occurred in 80 percent of the women with endometriosis, 70 percent of the women with severe menstrual pain, and 60 percent of the women with postoperative gynecological surgery.

Pycnogenol is spasmolytic (antispastic) and acts to reduce spasms of the uterus. The capillary-protecting activity of Pycnogenol may further contribute to soothe menstrual discomfort. Note, though, that Pycnogenol is not estrogen-mimicking.

Erectile Dysfunction (Impotence)

Erectile dysfunction (impotence) is a widespread problem affecting about 30 percent of men in their forties and about 67 percent of men in their seventies. In Chapter 4 we discussed nitric oxide and I mentioned its most vital role in the male penile erection. In order for erection to occur, additional blood must flow into the penis. The arteries supplying this blood depend on nitric oxide to allow them to relax and permit additional blood flow. This nitric oxide is made in the lining of the arteries by the enzyme nitric oxide synthase, using the amino acid arginine. Pycnogenol can stimulate the production of nitric oxide synthase and thus increase the production of the needed nitric oxide.

The erectile dysfunction drug sildenafil (Viagra) also works through a mechanism that increases nitric oxide production in these arteries. U.S. Patent No. 6,565,851 was issued on May 20, 2003, for the use of Pycnogenol in relieving symptoms of erectile dysfunction.

CHAPTER 11

ATTENTION DEFICIT DISORDERS (ADD AND ADHD)

Attention deficit disorder (ADD) and attention deficit hyperactivity disorder (ADHD) refer to a group of behavioral problems that used to be simply called "hyperactivity." They involve impulsive behavior, the inability to keep focused on a task, and/or hyperactivity.

The Causes of ADD and ADHD

The causes of ADD and ADHD are not known, but structural abnormalities have not been identified and at this time are believed not to be involved. The leading suspect appears to be problems with neurotransmitters, possibly associated with decreased activity or stimulation in the upper brain stem and frontal midbrain. There is also suspicion that toxins, environmental problems, or neurological immaturity could be causative factors.

How Pycnogenol Helps

One way Pycnogenol helps in ADD and ADHD is that the antioxidant effect of Pycnogenol keeps neurotransmitters functioning longer. Pycnogenol also improves circulation, including the microcirculation in the brain. The increased production of nitric oxide, which also acts as a neurotransmitter, may contribute to the improvement of memory and learning ability. However, I suspect that the effect of Pycnogenol is more complex than this. It will take more research to uncover exactly how Pycnogenol functions to help those with ADD or ADHD and to improve cognitive function in general.

Pycnogenol's Unexpected Benefit

I'll take credit for being the first to report this apparent benefit at a scientific meeting, but many individuals had already made the discovery, by accident, that Pycnogenol improved their ADD/ADHD symptoms. What regularly happens is that persons taking Pycnogenol for their hay fever will find that their ADD symptoms decrease within a week or two. Through the years, because I am the author of other books on Pycnogenol, I have received hundreds of letters reporting this.

I surveyed the case histories and experiences of several patients and found that Pycnogenol had helped all of the patients who tried it. I reported this small study at The Second International Pycnogenol Symposium in May 1995 in Biarritz, France.

In August 1995, I received a letter from psychologist Julie Paul, Ph.D., who told me that Pycnogenol had also helped her immensely, as well as her colleague, Dr. Stephen Tennebaum.

Studies

There are case reports in the medical literature, but I am not aware of any *large* clinical trials at this writing. A clinical trial involving thirty-six children will be discussed. One case report was described in the *Journal of the American Academy of Child & Adolescent Psychiatry* (1999; 38(4):357–358) by Dr. Steven Heimann of Evansville, Indiana.

Dr. Heimann tells of a child who was not responding well to drug therapy, but did respond well to the Pycnogenol given to him by his parents. Dr. Heimann studied the effects of Pycnogenol by taking the child off Pycnogenol and then reintroducing it. He reports, "The parents reluctantly agreed to give the child a trial off of Pycnogenol for four weeks to compare the effects of [drug] plus Pycnogenol to [drug] alone. Within two weeks of stopping Pycnogenol the patient became significantly more hyperactive and impulsive, marked by numerous demerits in school. He was also involved in several physical altercations, which previously had abated with Pycnogenol. The child's regimen of Pycnogenol was reinstated, and again he demonstrated significant improvement in ADHD target symptoms within three weeks."

In Japan, Dr. Hayashi Masao, a neurologist in Kani City, Gifu Prefecture, reported that Pycnogenol had a therapeutic effect in the treatment of ADHD symptoms in children. He concluded, "Although we still need more evidence of the effect of Pycnogenol in the treatment of ADHD, it is time to carry out the clinical trials to prove it." (Masao, H. Pycnogenol supplementation provides relief from ADHD symptoms in 70% of treated children. *Mainichi Shimbun* [Japan]. October 21, 2000.)

In Slovakia, researchers at Comenius University lead by Dr. J. Trebaticka gave thirty-six ADHD children 1 milligram of Pycnogenol per pound of body weight per day with good results. They concluded, "Our results show that one month of Pycnogenol administration causes a significant reduction of hyperactivity as evaluated by both teachers and parents. The children also demonstrated improved attention ability as measured objectively with standard psychological tests. In the placebo group, there was no improvement. One month after completing the study and the cessation of Pycnogenol, the children relapsed into hyperactivity." (Durackova, Z. et al.; published in *Polyphenols Communications;* Editors A. Hoikkala and O. Soidinsalo, Organic Chemistry Laboratory, University of Helsinki, Finland, printed by Gummerus Printing Jyväskylä, Finland, 2004.)

In a parallel study lead by Dr. Durackova Zdenka at the same University, it was determined that ADHD children had an increased amount of oxidized DNA. This may explain the mechanism through which the powerful antioxidant Pycnogenol works. They found, "Pycnogenol administration at one mg Pycnogenol per pound per day causes significant inhibition of oxidative damage to DNA and lowers adrenaline and noradrenaline levels." (Durackova, Z. et al., 2004.)

It is gratifying and reassuring to see these preliminary studies to verify Pycnogenol's positive effect on people with ADD and ADHD. Combined with my observations of this effect over a decade with hundreds of "anecdotal" reports, I believe it is time for a large-scale clinical trial. In the meantime, I will continue to recommend Pycnogenol for all forms of hyperactivity, including ADD and ADHD.

CHAPTER 12

How to Use Pycnogenol

If you are now convinced, as I am, that Pycnogenol may help you, you'll probably want some information on how to take it. This final chapter answers these practical, everyday questions. Select a manufacturer that you trust, determine the concentration suited for your purposes, and double-check to see if the label carries the Pycnogenol trademark (logo of a pine tree) or U.S. Patent No. 4,698,360, or mentions that it was produced by Horphag Research, Ltd. If none of these notations appear on the label, you may have an imitation, not Pycnogenol.

Determining the Amount for You

The correct dosage depends on why you wish to take Pycnogenol. If you just want to improve the synergistic effect of your nutritional antioxidants, you need only 20 to 25 milligrams of Pycnogenol a day. If you are seeking to optimize your antioxidant defenses, you may wish to take 50 to 100 milligrams a day. If you wish to protect your blood platelets from stress or smoke, or protect your eyes against retinopathy, or reduce the pain or swelling due to venous disorder, then you may need to take $1/2$ to 1 milligram for every pound of your body weight. As the condition improves, you may be able to start cutting this back to the 50 to 100 milligrams per day range.

It makes no practical difference in its absorption whether Pycnogenol is taken with meals or on an empty stomach. Pycnogenol rarely produces digestive disturbances, so it really doesn't matter when you take it. However, most people find that taking supplements with meals is easier, more convenient, and gentler on the system. Bioflavonoids, such as Pycnogenol, improve the absorption of vitamin C, so it is wise to take Pycnogenol with your other supplements.

As with vitamin C and other water-soluble nutrients, Pycnogenol is most effective when taken two or three times a day in divided doses. This maintains a constant level of Pycnogenol in the blood. However, there is no reason that your daily amount of Pycnogenol cannot be taken all at once. Note, though, that one Asian study reported that some persons became too active and could not sleep when they had taken the full dose of Pycnogenol in the evening.

Proven Safety

There is no known contraindication—that is, condition that would make treatment inadvisable—for Pycnogenol use. As always, pregnant women and small children should consult with their healthcare practitioner before taking any dietary supplement, herb, or medication. If your doctor has prescribed anticoagulants, you should ask him whether you might also use Pycnogenol, as it will also decrease the reactivity of blood platelets. The doctor may choose to recheck your blood-clotting time after you begin taking Pycnogenol along with your anti-coagulation medicine, and then lower the dosage of the anticoagulant if needed.

Millions of users regularly take Pycnogenol as a dietary supplement and to improve many health conditions. Pycnogenol has been in wide usage since the late 1960s with no reported serious adverse health effects. It has been studied by toxicologists who have concluded that Pycnogenol is safe.

Dozens and dozens of studies through the many years of use have shown that Pycnogenol is nontoxic, non-mutagenic (doesn't cause mutations in DNA), and noncarcinogenic (doesn't cause cancer). Studies also indicate that Pycnogenol will not cause birth defects, but I would never suggest that a woman of child-bearing age start taking any supplement without first checking with her physician.

Dr. Peter Rohdewald has overseen safety studies of Pycnogenol since 1982. He is a pharmaceutical researcher and teaches pharmaceutical science. He is well versed in toxicology and the safety of nutrients and drugs and has served as the Commissarial Director of the Institute for Pharmaceutical Chemistry at the University of Munster.

Several acute toxicity studies found that it would take 336 grams—nearly 1 pound—of Pycnogenol to cause any type of toxic effects in a 155-pound person. Studies of long-term toxicity found that adverse effects would not be produced until 11,250 milligrams of Pycnogenol a day were taken for more than six months by a 150-pound person. The highest recommended dose of Pycnogenol is about 360 milligrams a day in studies on venous disorders. There were no side effects. More typical dosages would be in the 50 to 100 milligrams per day range. Pycnogenol is safe as a daily food supplement when taken as recommended.

Pycnogenol is "generally recognized as safe" (GRAS). A panel of independent toxicology experts reviewed the toxicology data on Pycnogenol for the U.S. Food and Drug Administration (FDA). According to a leading safety expert, Dr. George Burdock (a member of the American Board of Toxicology), the available safety data on Pycnogenol are so numerous and compelling that the GRAS status of Pycnogenol was achieved with ease. Pycnogenol has not only been well tested for safety in animal studies, but the tolerance in humans is also well documented. The known body of scientific evidence confirms that Pycnogenol can safely be taken daily throughout life.

CONCLUSION

By now, you understand why Pycnogenol has excited so many people. It can help protect you from a variety of diseases—including various types of heart disease and circulatory disorders—aggravated by free radicals. It can boost your immune system and help protect you from infectious diseases.

As scientists have become interested in Pycnogenol, they have been motivated to investigate and discover its specific and highly detailed mechanisms. They are learning how Pycnogenol interacts with nitric oxide, cellular adhesion molecules, and many other biochemical molecules.

In review, Pycnogenol is a very powerful natural antioxidant that should be consumed daily to protect the body against the harmful free radicals that cause degenerative and age-related diseases. Pycnogenol reduces the risk of heart attacks and strokes. Pycnogenol restores blood platelets to their normal condition and reduces the stickiness that can lead to heart attacks and stroke.

Pycnogenol protects the inner lining of blood vessels. Pycnogenol also supports healthy blood pressure and normalizes healthy cholesterol levels.

Pycnogenol helps improve circulation by relaxing the constriction of arteries and other blood vessels that is caused by the stress hormones adrenaline and noradrenaline. Thus, Pycnogenol has an antistress function supporting a better blood flow during periods of stressful living.

Pycnogenol binds to collagen in the skin to

maintain skin elasticity, helping to keep skin firm and reduce wrinkles. Pycnogenol also improves microcirculation of the tiny skin capillaries, supporting better oxygen and nutrient supply and better hydration as well as protecting against sun damage. Pycnogenol usage over time can result in fewer wrinkles and smoother skin with a healthy and vibrant glow and tone.

Pycnogenol is of special value to diabetics in reducing diabetic retinopathy and cataracts.

In writing about Pycnogenol over the years and frequently talking with scientists who do the actual research on this remarkable substance, I have continued to be impressed by its positive effects on health. Obviously, I take it myself, and perhaps not surprisingly, I am convinced that everyone could benefit from Pycnogenol supplements.

SELECTED
REFERENCES

Araghi-Nicknam, M., Hosseini, S., Larson D., Rohdewald, P., and Watson R.R. Pine bark extract reduces platelet aggregation. *Integrative Medicine*, 1999; 2(2/3):73–77.

Arcangeli, P. Pycnogenol in chronic venous insufficiency. *Fitoterapia*, 2000; 71:236–244.

Bayeta, E., and Lau, B.H.S. Pycnogenol inhibits generation of inflammatory mediators in the macrophages. *Nutrition Res.*, 1999; 20:249–259.

Belcaro, G., Cesarone, M.R., Rohdewald, P., et al. Prevention of venous thrombosis and thrombophlebitis in long-haul flights with Pycnogenol. *Clin. Appl. Thrombosis/Hemostasis*, 2004; 10(4):T1–T10.

Durackova, Z. et al. The effect of Pycnogenol on the Erythrocyte Membrane Fluidity. *Gen. Physiol. Biophys*, 2004; 23: 39–51.

Fitzpatrick, D.F., Bing, B., and Rohdewald, P. Endothelium-dependent vascular effects of Pycnogenol. *Journal Cardiovascular Pharmacology*, 1998; 32:509–515.

Gulati, O.P. Pycnogenol in venous disorders: A review. *European Bulletin of Drug Research*, 1999; 7(2):8–13.

Hosseini et al. A randomized, double-blind, placebo-controlled, prospective, 16 week crossover study to determine the role of Pynogenol in modifying blood pressure in mildly hypertensive patients. *Nutrition Research*, 2001; 21:1251–1260.

Kohama, T., and Suzuki, N. The treatment of gynaecological disorders with Pycnogenol. *European Bulletin of Drug Research*, 1999; 7(2):30–32.

Kohama, T., Suzuki, N., Satoshi, O., and Inoue, M. Analgesic efficacy of French maritime pine extract in dysmenorrhea: An open clinical trial. *J. Reprod. Med.*, 2004; 49(10):828–31.

Liu, F., Zhang, Y., and Lau, B.H.S. Pycnogenol improves learning impairment and memory deficit in senescence-accelerated mice. *Journal of Anti-aging Medicine*, 1999; 2(4):349–355.

Liu, X., Wei, J., Tan, F., et al. Antidiabetic effect of Pycnogenol French maritime pine bark extract in patients with diabetes type II. *Life Sciences,* 2004; 75:2505–13.

Packer, L., Rimbach, G., and Virgili, F. Antioxidant activity and biologic properties of a procyanidin-rich extract from the pine (*Pinus maritima*) bark, Pycnogenol. Review article in *Free Radical Biology and Medicine,* 1999; 27(5/6): 704–724.

Pavlovic, P. Improved endurance by use of antioxidants. *European Bulletin of Drug Research,*1999; 7(2):26–29.

Petrassi, C., Mastromarino, A., and Spartera, C. Pycnogenol in chronic venous insufficiency. *Phytomedicine,* 2000; 7(5):383–388.

Pütter, M., Grotemeyer, K.H.M., Würthwein, G., Araghi-Nicknam, M., Watson, R.R., Hosseini, S., and Rohdewald, P. Inhibition of smoking-induced platelet aggregation by aspirin and Pycnogenol. *Thrombosis Research,* 1999; 95:155–161.

Rohdewald, P. A review of the French maritime pine bark extract (Pycnogenol®), a herbal medication with a diverse clinical pharmacology. *International Journal of Clinical Pharmacology and Therapeutics,* 2002; 40(4): 158–168.

Roseff, J. Improvement in sperm quality and function with French maritime pine tree bark extract. *The Journal of Reproductive Medicine,* 2002; 47:821–824.

Saliou, C., Rimbach, G., Moini, H., McLaughlin, L., Hosseini, S., Lee, J., Watson, R.R., and Packer, L. Solar ultraviolet-induced erythema in human skin and nuclear factor-kappa-B-dependent gene expression in keratinocytes are modulated by a French maritime pine bark extract. *Free Radical Biology and Medicine,* 2001; 30(2):154–160.

Sharma, S.C., Sharma, S. and Gulati, O. Pycnogenol® inhibits the release of histamine from mast cells. *Phytotherapy Research* 17(1) 66–69.

Sime, S., and Reeve, V.E. Protection from inflammation, immunosuppression and carcinogenesis induced by UV radiation in mice by topical Pycnogenol. *Photochem. & Photobiol.,* 2003; 79(2):8655.

Spadea, L., and Balestrazzi, E. Treatment of vascular retinopathies with Pycnogenol. *Phytotherapie Research,* 2001; 15:1–5.

Watson, R. Pycnogenol and cardiovascular health. *Evidenced-Based Integrative Medicine,* 2003; 1:27–32.

OTHER RESOURCES

Helpful Websites about Pycnogenol
www.pycnogenol.com
www.drpasswater.com

GreatLife Magazine
Consumer magazine with articles on vitamins, minerals, herbs, and foods.

Available for free at many health and natural food stores.

Let's Live Magazine
Consumer magazine with emphasis on the health benefits of vitamins, minerals, and herbs.

Customer service:
1-800-676-4333
P.O. Box 74908
Los Angeles, CA 90004

Subscriptions: 12 issues per year, $19.95 in the U.S.; $31.95 outside the U.S.

Physical Magazine
Magazine oriented to body builders and other serious athletes.

Customer service:
1-800-676-4333
P.O. Box 74908
Los Angeles, CA 90004

Subscriptions: 12 issues per year, $19.95 in the U.S.; $31.95 outside the U.S.

The Nutrition Reporter™ newsletter

Monthly newsletter that summarizes recent medical research on vitamins, minerals, and herbs.

Customer service:

P.O. Box 30246

Tucson, AZ 85751-0246

e-mail: jack@thenutritionreporter.com

www.nutritionreporter.com

Subscriptions: $26 per year (12 issues) in the U.S.; $32 U.S. or $48 CNC for Canada; $38 for other countries

INDEX